Dementia
HOME CARE

How to Prepare
Before, During, and After

TRACY CRAM PERKINS

Behler
PUBLICATIONS
USA

Behler Publications

Dementia Home Care
A Behler Publications Book

Copyright © 2021 by Tracy Cram Perkins
Cover design by Yvonne Parks - www.pearcreative.ca
Back cover photography by Mark Bennington
Recipes by Cathy Russell

Some names have been changed to protect their privacy.

Library of Congress Cataloging-in-Publication Data
Names: Perkins, Tracy Cram, author.
Title: Dementia home care : how to prepare before, during, and after /
  Tracy Cram Perkins.
Description: Lake Jackson : Behler Publications, [2021] | Includes
  bibliographical references and index. | Summary: "Comprehensive A-Z
  examination of the role of care giver for Alzheimer's/Dementia patients
  that offers help with making informed decisions about in-home care
  giving"-- Provided by publisher.
Identifiers: LCCN 2020052025 (print) | LCCN 2020052026 (ebook) | ISBN
  9781941887127 (paperback) | ISBN 9781941887134 (epub)
Subjects: LCSH: Dementia--Patients--Care. | Alzheimer's disease. |
  Dementia--Patients--Family relationships.
Classification: LCC RC521 .P4245 2021 (print) | LCC RC521 (ebook) | DDC
  616.8/31--dc23
LC record available at https://lccn.loc.gov/2020052025
LC ebook record available at https://lccn.loc.gov/2020052026

Print ISBN: 9781941887127
Ebook ISBN: 9781941887134

Dedication

This book is dedicated to my father, Eldon, who taught me how to rebuild my first car, who taught me how to fish, who could never convince me vanilla ice cream was the ultimate flavor because you secretly loved strawberry, and who continued to teach me up to the very end. Thank you for the time you spent with me and for asking the question, "I have Alzheimer's, not the plague. What will it take to be treated like a human being? That's all I'm asking."

Acknowledgments

My beta readers, Johanna Flynn, Lisa Knight, Julie Cooper, Sharon Jackson, Venetia Runnion, Wendy Kendall, Andrea Ball, Cathy Russell, Karen Munger, Vickie Barrier, Indy Quillen, Debi Canales, Steve Wilkendorf, Lori Ann Nelsen-Allen, Teri Choate, Lindsay Pierce, Nancy Conway, and Debbie Moffett, your input made this book what it is today. Without your help this book would not have been possible.

The Lodge Ladies: Andrea Finchum, Gail Galloway, Kim Governor-Sproul, Susan Hamilton Wolfe, Wendy Jackson, and Nancy Forst English for your unwavering support. Kristina Younger for her lifetime support. Matt Hawkins and Eli Hawkins for sharing the caregiving. Gail Cram for her sisterly support and suggestions. My sister, Sandy Murphy, for being my biggest cheerleader. Beverly Cram for being with me through it all for her little brother.

Shereé Landers for the tips on treating hypothermia. Vanessa Palensky for tips on distraction techniques. Ursula Nicol for tips using the warm blankets.

Thank you, Lynn Price, my editor, for your faith and support on this project.

To the women who taught me and inspired me through their books and videos: Jolene Brackey, Joanne Koenig Coste, Paula Spencer Scott, and Teepa Snow.

To my husband, Daniel, who shared this journey with me, who inspired me to write these pages, and who gave me the emotional support to cross the finish line. You are my once in a lifetime.

Table of Contents

Chapter 1: Introduction

We all look for quick answers and shortcuts. Especially when we are under great stress. This book is for anyone who is struggling to care for someone with dementia. It contains what-can-I-try-in-this-moment tips you can use whether you are caring for your family member or friend.

Each person's journey is different. The road of dementia care will change every aspect of your life and theirs. Dementia is like playing Hide and Seek: "Ready or not, *here I come.*"

None of us saw dementia barreling down the hill at us like a Mack truck with no brakes, because it arrived slowly with plausible explanations for everything. Only when we look back do we see the mounting evidence.

No two people experience dementia the same way. No two family members will care for a loved one with dementia the same way. Caring for someone with dementia is one of the most stressful burdens a person can ever accept. We have more training to drive a car, operate a smart phone, or boil water than we do to take care of someone who is saying the long goodbye.

Unlike a day job, with dementia care there are no vacations, no pay raises, no glowing performance reviews. Unlike raising a child, there is no first day of kindergarten, no graduations, no weddings to look forward to.

My journey started when my younger sister called to tell me our father reached his tipping point and didn't have the health to continue caring for our mother. Our mother had cancer and the treatment caused her dementia. My husband and I decided I would quit my job and take over my mother's care. What I didn't know then was my father already traveled down the road of Alzheimer's Disease. Alzheimer's Disease is a great mimic, disguising itself as anything else, even from the person who has the disease. I didn't discover he had *it* for several more years.

I wasn't a caregiver. I didn't know the first thing about caregiving. I didn't have any medical training. I did know I needed help and lots of it.

The caregiver, that's you—and me. You may think a caregiver is a person working at a skilled nursing facility who is trained and gets paid. Nope, we fall into the category. We tend to think of ourselves as wives, husbands, life partners, daughters, sons, friends, or extended family. You are a caregiver. Even if you're three thousand miles away and managing as much as humanly possible over the phone, you are still a caregiver. We are America's largest health care provider, the unpaid family caregivers.

Dementia care is difficult. It requires patience, adaptability, and a strong back. From learning how to transfer someone who doesn't want a bath in and out of a tub to dealing with verbal abuse caused by delusions and paranoia. As the caregiver of my family, I know firsthand the depression and anxiety and guilt which comes with dementia care.

My biggest frustrations occurred when something happened with my father and I would vaguely remember reading about ways to take care of the issue but couldn't find it in any of the books on my bookshelf. Days after the event I would find the possible solutions when I was looking for something else. This book grew from not being able to find the information that should have been at the end of my tired, stressed-out fingertips.

I have organized this book with emphasis on the caregiver. Not everyone with dementia will present symptoms in the same order. The chapters are ordered with the general progression of the disease. In this way, you won't spend a lot of time searching for help, instead, you will spend a little time finding possible workable solutions.

Unlike other books in this arena, the chapter on laughter is at the front of this book. You will find it is one of the best tools in your toolbox. Not enough attention is paid to the therapeutic effects of laughter.[1, 2, 3] My husband and I found the easiest ways to motivate my father involved joyous laughter. We made sure it was one of the last things he heard before he passed.

"Laughter is not at all a bad beginning for a friendship, and it is far the best ending for one." -Oscar Wilde

Clarification of Terms

You will notice when you read this book, I describe the person affected by dementia or more specifically Alzheimer's as a loved one. After this chapter, I will use the term loved one sparingly. I realize not every caregiving situation is with someone you love. It could be an estranged spouse, one of your cantankerous in-laws, stepsiblings, or someone whose lifestyle you didn't agree with. We don't use the snappy words *caree or carer* here yet like they do in the U.K. What I will do is vary by chapter using the pronouns she or he or they after the introduction of the word loved one. In most cases, however, the majority of people who receive the caregiving are cared for by people who love them.

How This Book Works

This book is designed for reading from start to finish or fanning through the pages until you find what you are searching for. Each chapter contains a text box listing the content of the chapter. For those of you happier with a table of contents or an index, you will find them at the front and rear of this book. For those of you reading from start to finish, you may notice some repetition of subject matter in several chapters. This is for the active page fanner who otherwise might miss an important tidbit.

Within some of the chapters are text boxes listing suggested materials for activities, explanation of terms, or possible solutions to an issue you may be experiencing with your loved one where applicable.

For example, your mother tells you, "The animal drank go juice." What is she trying to say?

In the chapter *Memory Aids and the Family,* you will find the <u>Five Magic Words and More</u>[4] with a text box listing questions you can ask her in conjunction with using cue cards that may clear up what she is saying. It could be she wants more coffee with her breakfast, or she thinks the dog needs to go outside for a personal moment.

> **The Five Magic Words and More Phrases**
> - Tell me more about XXX?
> - Describe a/an XXX for me?
> - Show me a/an XXX?
> - Show me what XXX does?
> - Show me how you use it?

I encourage you to write down a special or humorous moment with your loved one or jot down notes in a journal. In the chapter *The Power of Laughter; The Caregiver's Perspective,* page 7, I share an example from my own journal to give you an idea how to get started if you are not used to journaling. Writing it down will help manage your stress and give you a cherished keepsake once you have recovered from caregiving.

The Appendices contain further examples referenced in various chapters and footnote citations, along with information on where to get additional materials, including websites and suggested reading.

Now let's get on with your journey.

†Some of the names of the caregivers in the anecdotes have been changed.

Chapter 2: The Power of Laughter; the Caregiver's Perspective

"Laugh (n). A smile that burst." ~John Donovan

A Good Laugh a Day Soothes Tension Away

If you are reading this, someone you care about has some form of dementia. For family members and caregivers, dementia will change every aspect of their lives.

Whether they live in a different state and call regularly or are sharing a home with a loved one, the situation will be stressful.

When it happened to me, I didn't realize I was already a caregiver, driving my dad to doctor's appointments, helping him with meal preparations. I didn't realize I would need a crash course in everything from administering medications to working through hallucinations. I didn't realize it wasn't about me. It was about my dad.

I needed to slow down to enter the Alzheimer's "school zone."

Typical example: After dinner, my father opened the refrigerator door and rummaged around. He found a block of white cheddar cheese in one of the keepers. He opened the package and took a huge bite from the cheese block.

I walked into the kitchen to wash the dinner dishes. My father's cheeks bulged; his mouth partially open.

"Dad, what are you doing?" My voice rose half an octave and my blood pressure rode the elevator through the ceiling.

He glared at me and put his empty hand on his hip. "I'm hungry," he said. His mouth full of cheese. A piece of cheese flew from his mouth to the floor.

He finished half the block and placed it back in the fridge. Leaving the refrigerator door open, he wandered to his bedroom.

Something needed to change, and he couldn't change. The progression of the disease meant change could only go in one direction. It was up to me. I needed to laugh.

Let's put this into perspective. Hold your hand up in front of your face. Place your palm against the tip of your nose. What can you see? Could you walk around without bumping into things? Maybe. You can see around the outside of your hand, just not what's right in front of you. Your vision is limited, isolated. That's what caregiving for someone with dementia does. It isolates. It exhausts. It depresses.

Move your hand out a foot from your nose. This is where you are with a good support network. It's a place of safety, respite, sharing, caring, isolation relieving. A place to ask for help. <u>Don't isolate yourself</u>. Support comes in many forms, accept the gift that it offers. Not everyone will ask for help or will have the time to join a support group—even one online. For your own well-being, I urge you to join one.

Move your hand out to arm's length. This is where a laugh a day drives the tension away. If you don't laugh, dementia's side effects will put up roadblocks with the strength of amorous skunks on a hot August afternoon. Who wants that?

Laughter's Health Benefits[5]

You cannot laugh without being present in the moment. It will lower your tension, your blood pressure, loosen your muscles, boost your immune system, and release those wonderful endorphins which are natural pain killers and mood enhancers—for free, no prescription necessary.

Laughter Inducing Techniques

Dr. Annette Goodheart, a pioneer in the field of laughter therapy, practiced in Santa Barbara, California, during her lifetime. She referred to laughter as "Portable therapy." She wrote, *Laughter Therapy, How to Laugh About Everything in Your Life That Isn't Really Funny,* encompassing her experiences and the benefits of laughing.

In the chapter titled, "The Big Tee Hee," Dr. Goodheart said, "We are taught in this culture to face our problems straight on, to be brave, and to strive to solve those problems, not avoid them or skirt the issues. We all want to do the right thing, and so we try hard to solve our problems as our culture has taught us—head on, directly, and with great seriousness. This approach is often paralyzing. It is remarkable that we do as well as we do under these circumstances."

Give yourself permission to laugh and to cry.

If you have difficulty laughing, use one of Dr. Goodheart's examples. Say out loud the issue that is bothering you and follow it with the words, "Tee Hee."

For example, "My mother doesn't remember me, tee hee."

Repeat it.

Repeat it again.

If it doesn't work, up the ante at the end of the sentence and say, "My mother doesn't remember me, heh, heh."

You will laugh because you feel ridiculous and your shoulders may loosen. Schedule Tee-Hee coffee klatches and practice with a friend. You need a good laugh, maybe even a good guffaw. Heh, heh.

You need to release the emotions, tension, stress, or you'll run out of life before your loved one.

When you laugh, also belly laugh with your loved one. She may be confused, but she will laugh too, and everyone's mood will be elevated. For example, Vickie, a member of ACT III, a volunteer organization for people in the third act of their lives, shared a recent experience from the first time she met someone with dementia.

> *"Until recently I really hadn't been exposed to many people suffering from dementia. My friend's 98-year-old mother is suffering dementia, although not Alzheimer's. She doesn't remember where she is or where she's going. When she asks, her daughter laughs while reminding her. Then the mother laughs too. Until that experience, I would have become irritated and snappish. Now, what would that have accomplished?"*

Look for the humor in situations that arise because of dementia. Your loved one may do or say some very funny things. Be sure you're laughing with them and not at them.

My father and I used to sing nursery rhymes together. He could not remember the words to the last line of "Pop! Goes the Weasel" and it morphed into "Poop goes the noodle." We laughed every time.

Watch comedies together; your regular life is filled with enough drama already.

If you have young children in your life, take the time to enjoy their laughter. Make it a multi-generational event. Laughing children are infectious. Catch the laughter, share the laughter, spend your laughter like it's going out of style.

After your loved one goes to bed or is wandering the halls because of Sundowners (a worsening of behaviors in the evening, see *Distraction Techniques*, Page 102), watch a late-night talk show or subscribe to an internet joke service that matches your taste and humor. If you have cable, watch Comedy Central.

On those days when you won't allow yourself to cry, laugh into your pillow, or in the shower.

The Surgeon General's warning for laughter could read, "Warning, laughter produces chemicals known to the State of California to be cathartic and to make you feel better. Other states of mind may follow." Hee, hee, hee.

Suggestions for Using a Journal

One of the best tools I discovered while taking care of my father was journaling the humorous or special moments we shared during the day. It helped me keep my sanity and my sense of humor.

For example, my husband, Daniel, and I took my father on road trips almost every weekend until he became too ill to travel. One weekend we chose the town of Leavenworth, Washington, because it has special significance for my family.

My Journal Entry

"*My mother was born in Leavenworth, and my great grandparents owned a card room there during prohibition. My great grandmother swore until the day she died they only sold soft drinks.*

My grandfather's photo album entitled, "Me and It" shows bottles and cases of liquor being received in the back country and secreted into town.

Because of the card room, every member of my family learned a variation of the card game "Canfield" played by the high rollers. The variation we play is called "Demon" and my dad and I play almost every day at lunch. How well he plays lets me know what kind of an evening we are going to have.

Before we left for Leavenworth, I handed my dad his overcoat, hat, and gloves. He set his coat and gloves on top of my car and put on his hat while I climbed into the middle of the bench seat in the Love Wagon (a red, Ford F150). He climbed in next to me. Daniel was already behind the wheel.

I'm not a morning person, so I didn't notice until over 2 hours later when we arrived in Leavenworth that he didn't have his coat or gloves. It was snowing and 31°F (-1°C) outside.

My dad was very upset he forgot his coat and gloves and his mood darkened.

We walked into a clothing store on the main street at the west end of town. Near the front entrance stood three racks of various style gloves. I asked my dad to try on a pair.

He said, "I know how to fix this Tracy." He walked over to the counter where a tall, smiling, middle-aged, frosted-blond woman stood behind the cash register.

He smiled at the woman. He said loudly, "I've got big hands," while holding his hands six inches from her face, making fists then opening his hands to emphasize each word.

He repeated himself two more times before she recovered enough to figure out he needed help with gloves.

She linked her arm in one of his and they walked over to the first display rack. She said, "I believe I have the perfect gloves for you."

She handed my father a pair of tan wool gloves with brown leather padding on the fingers and palms.

He put them on his hands and sighed loudly. He held up his hands and flexed his fingers for everyone to see. His shit-eating grin said it all."

There is just something about "I've got big hands," which puts a big smile on my face. He's been gone for a while now, but I still go back and re-read it and laugh out loud.

Take the time to write down those special moments. It may help you laugh while you relive the moment. You will appreciate it even more when your loved one is gone.

Laughing in a Public Restroom

If you don't think you've got a reason to laugh, remember my initials are T.P. For the rest of your life you will remember me every time you run out of toilet paper and write my initials on your grocery list or when you're in the bathroom after your morning constitutional.

It happened to me in a public restroom shortly after I married my husband. We dined in a restaurant in Newport, Oregon. I excused myself for the call of nature. While I was ruminating, my new initials flashed across my brain-scape like a movie marquee. The more I thought about my new initials the more I laughed. It's amazing how fast the room clears when someone belly laughs in one of the restroom stalls.

If you can laugh, you can survive caregiving.

But if you're in a public restroom and you think of me and laugh out loud, you're on your own.

Chapter 3: What is Dementia and Alzheimer's Disease and What isn't?

"Unless we remember, we cannot understand."
~E.M. Forster

We all have moments of distraction or forgetfulness that are not dementia. Occasionally putting the milk in the cupboard and the cereal in the refrigerator are normal. Forgetting how to change the settings on the television with the remote and needing some help is normal.

Forgetting what day of the week it is and remembering later is normal. Forgetting where the bathroom is in your apartment is not. Occasionally forgetting someone's name is normal. If you notice your loved one is pausing longer and longer during sentences searching for a word, not normal.

Memory loss is not dementia. While it is a symptom of dementia, there are several other symptoms which need to be present for a dementia diagnosis.

Not everyone with dementia will become aggressive. Aggression, in general, is activated by the way someone is treated or communicated with and not a symptom of dementia by itself.

- Dementia is a symptom of something, not a diagnosis of a disease.
- Dementia is not a normal part of aging.
- Dementia is a loss of mental powers severe enough to interfere with daily living.

It's not Old Man Snodgrass cussing out CNN or telling you what he thinks of your haircut. He's probably an old grump.

A diagnosis of dementia does not mean someone's life is over. Even though the condition is progressive there are many strategies and treatments available to help make life as full and rich as possible for many years to come.

It is also common for people diagnosed with dementia to have mixed dementia. According to the National Institute on Aging, mixed dementia is a combination of two or more types of dementia. Any number of combinations is possible, for example a person can have Alzheimer's disease and vascular dementia. It is another reason why no two people with dementia will react or progress the same way.

Everyone with dementia does not end up in a nursing home, or you wouldn't be reading this book.

Other Types of Dementia Defined

Dementia is a broad umbrella term, not a single disease, and while Alzheimer's Disease is the most common type of dementia, there are over 90 other types.

Some of the less common types of dementia include:

- Frontotemporal Dementia (FTD), such as Pick's Disease, a progressive form of dementia which occurs in middle age, often runs in families, and causes localized shrinkage of the brain
- Korsakoff's Disease which is alcohol related
- Parkinson's Dementia and Lewy Body Dementia, a type of progressive dementia that damages brain cells over time because of abnormal microscopic deposits, may be linked
- Creutzfeldt-Jakob Disease (CJD) is fatal and linked to infectious prion proteins in the brain; most cases occur spontaneously and cannot be spread without direct contact to brain or spinal tissue
- HIV-associated dementia (HAD)
- Vascular dementia caused by strokes

Alzheimer's Disease (A.D.) is a disease for which, at the time of this writing, there is no known cause, is no cure, and is fatal. More than 75 percent of people with dementia have Alzheimer's Disease.[6]

When we talk about something dementia related it will also relate to A.D. When we talk about something that is A.D. related, it may not apply to dementia.

The appearance of conditions attributed to dementia or A.D. can sometimes be caused by other medical conditions, for example:

- Poorly managed diabetes
- Drug interactions (prescription, over the counter, and/or illicit/recreational drugs)
- Infection
- Alcohol abuse
- Depression or mental health issues
- Dehydration
- Poor nutrition (such as a vitamin imbalance)
- Trauma (physical or emotional)
- Metabolic disorder
- Thyroid issues

> **Metabolic disorder** is a group of conditions that occur together, increasing the risk of heart disease, stroke, and type 2 diabetes. It also includes increased high blood pressure, high blood sugar, excess body fat around the waist, and abnormal cholesterol or triglyceride levels.

- Brain tumors
- Recent application of general anesthetic in a medical/surgical procedure
- Anticholinergic medications,* including habitual use of over-the-counter (OTC) sleep aids (Nyquil, Tylenol PM, among others), Benadryl, antidepressants, anti-heartburn medications such as Prilosec or Nexium and drugs taken specifically for Parkinson's Disease. Studies indicate that taking many of these drugs long-term may raise the risk of developing dementia by 30 percent.[7, 8]

Anticholinergic medications are a broad class of medications that are used to treat various medical conditions which involve both contraction and relaxation of muscles.

If these issues are untreated, they can cause irreparable damage, both physical and emotional and even death. If treated some of these disorders can be cured, unlike A.D.

Clinicians are using the MMSE (Mini Mental State Exam) to screen for dementia. It is now being used more often with the VAT (Visual Associative Test) which uses pictorial cue cards to evaluate associative memory. Adding the VAT to the evaluation process increases the accuracy of predicting dementia in patients. This kind of brief screening by a trained physician can help medical care providers and family caregivers plan for the person's needs now and in the future.[9]

Only a medical professional can properly diagnose if the symptoms are dementia and what the root cause may be. The evaluation will include a physical exam, a complete medical history, which includes hospitalizations, family history of illnesses, causes of death, drug interaction checks, nutrition consultation, and other possible causes. There may be a psychological and/or neurological exam as well.

What is Alzheimer's Disease

Alzheimer's Disease is a type of dementia that causes problems with memory, thinking, and behavior. Symptoms usually develop slowly and get worse over time, becoming severe enough to interfere with daily tasks.

According to the Alzheimer's Association the disease has ten warning signs:

- Loss of memory that disrupts daily life
- Challenges in planning or solving problems
- Difficulty completing familiar tasks at home, at work, or at leisure
- Confusion with time or place
- Trouble understanding visual images and spatial relationships
- New problems with words in speaking or writing
- Misplacing things and losing the ability to retrace steps
- Decreased or poor judgment

- Withdrawal from work or social activities
- Changes in mood and personality

Activities of Daily Living

Medical professionals and social workers who work with aging populations will want to know about your loved one's Activities of Daily Living (ADL) or Basic Activities of Daily Living (BADL). ADL's are walking, eating, dressing, grooming, toileting, bathing, and transferring, for example being able to move one's body from a bed to a chair.

In addition, your loved one will be assessed for their self-care tasks called Instrumental Activities of Daily Living (IADL). These include managing finances, managing transportation, like driving or other means, shopping for groceries, cooking, house cleaning and home maintenance, answering the telephone, handling mail, and managing their medications.

ADL's and IADL's are used to assess your loved one's condition. Can they walk around their home safely, feed themselves, dress by themselves? Can they clean their home, pay their bills, prepare a meal, and manage their medications? Knowing your loved one's ADL's and IADL's helps with planning the level of care. It will make it easier for you to monitor changes to what is happening with your loved one over time. It will also make it easier for your geriatrician(s) (medical professionals who work with older adults) to assess where you might be having difficulties managing their care without help.

Once you have gathered this information, you will be able to include it in your loved one's daily routine list which we will discuss in the chapter *Emergency Preparedness* on page 47.

Stages of the Disease

In most cases, Alzheimer's Disease progresses slowly, but not always. The symptoms worsen over time. A person with A.D. can live from four to twenty years after the diagnosis.

Alzheimer's Disease typically follows three general stages, which are mild cognitive impairment, moderate cognitive impairment, and severe cognitive impairment.

Mild cognitive impairment is the early-stage or early-onset of the disease. The person with mild impairment can still function with independence. They can still drive and be part of social activities. However, they will feel like they are having memory lapses, such as forgetting everyday objects or familiar words. They need to rely on memory aids such as reminder notes or electronic devices to keep themselves on track.

Family, friends, and co-workers will begin to notice the difficulties the person with mild impairment is experiencing.

In this stage, they may have problems remembering the right word or name, forgetting recently learned information, or have challenges performing tasks in social or work settings. They may forget material that they just read or misplace valuable objects such as keys or important documents and not be able to retrace their steps.

Moderate cognitive impairment (MCI) is, in most cases, the longest stage of the disease. It can last for many years. At this point, the person with MCI will require a greater level of care.

Symptoms will become very noticeable. You may notice the person with MCI's words getting confused, or they become angry or frustrated or act in unexpected ways, such as flushing garbage down the toilet, not remembering they just ate and demanding more food, or refusing to bathe.

They will forget portions of their own personal history or events they participated in and invent a new personal history. Many times, the new history is based on something they just heard or saw on television. They may forget family members and relationships, including spouses, adult children, and grandchildren. This can be especially painful. They may also add to their personal history by embellishing stories, going on in detail about trips they've never taken, imagining romantic relationships that never existed, and oversharing personal information or act out in sexually inappropriate ways.

They won't remember what their street address is or their telephone number or where they went to school. Their sleep patterns may invert such as sleeping during the day and being restless at night (See *Distraction Techniques*, page 91). They will become moody and withdraw from social interactions. Some individuals will have issues controlling their bowels and bladder.

This is the stage where they are most at risk for wandering off and becoming lost (See *Preparing Your Living Environment for Your Loved One*, page 71). They may also experience a personality change, such as becoming suspicious or delusional, or exhibit repetitive behavior like picking at their skin or clothing or wringing their hands.

In the final stage of the disease, Severe Cognitive Impairment, also known as late-stage Alzheimer's Disease, they will not be able to respond to their environment. Their ability to carry on a conversation will end and eventually they won't be able to control their own movements. They may still be able to say words or short phrases, but they will no longer be able to communicate pain.

At this stage, they may need round-the-clock assistance for every activity including personal care. They will lose physical abilities such as the ability to walk, sit, and swallow. They may even curl into a fetal position. They will lose awareness of any recent experience. At this stage they may become susceptible to infections, like pneumonia, which is most commonly caused by inhaling food into their lungs when they swallow.

Not every person with A.D. will present symptoms in the order described above. Because every person is different, how they react to the disease will be different. Some may experience difficulties swallowing in the moderate stage ahead of the late stage. Others may lose bowel and bladder control during the end of the mild stage.

The stages are a guideline used to assess where an individual is within the progression of the disease.

Knowing Your Own Limitations Before You Make the Decision for Care

Caregiving isn't easy, especially when you're dealing with an adult who is experiencing cognitive decline and behavioral changes brought on by dementia. In time you will need to deal with the difficult issues of incontinence, behavior control, and other debilities. But it can also be rewarding, especially when your patience learns to run an ultramarathon. Your view of the world will change for the better.

Not everyone is cut out to be a caregiver and that is all right. There are other ways to be supportive to your loved one.

More than likely, you have a job outside the home, children, and a household to run. You might not even live in the same city, state, or time zone. You may have multiple family members with strong or varied opinions about the best course of action.

If you are considering becoming the caregiver for your loved one, remember they will no longer be the person you remember. The loss of that connection can be devastating. You may want the help of a counselor, minister, or therapist who can help you cope with the loss. Learn to recognize your flash points, so the normal pressures and tension of caregiving don't spill over into anger. Consider writing down your hot buttons triggered by your loved one and then figure out a way to diffuse your response and possibly modify your loved one's behavior (See *The Power of Laughter; The Caregiver's Perspective*, page 4).

Taking care of a spouse takes a deeper, more intimate, emotional toll. If you are caring for a spouse, it can be more difficult to get time out or connect with friends or even relatives. You are at even greater risk for depression. Visit the Well Spouse Association at www.wellspouse.org. They are a non-profit and have local chapters around the country who offer face-to-face support groups. They also offer local phone support for spouses with partners who have a chronic illness—like dementia, and disabilities. If you cannot connect with a support group, vent your feelings on paper. Keep a journal to keep your sanity.

Consider a group caregiving option. Group care consists of a bunch of friends, family, co-workers or anyone else you know who would volunteer to help care for your loved one and you and your family, so that no one single person must bear the brunt of the caregiving. ShareTheCaregiving, Inc. is a non-profit centered around the book *Share the Care, How to Organize a Group to Care for Someone who is Seriously Ill*. They crafted their program to lead friends, neighbors, co-workers, and even acquaintances with a guided plan for creating and maintaining a 'caregiving family' to support someone they know facing a health, aging, medical issue—including dementia, or any circumstance where support is needed. The program covers every aspect of caregiving, including the tight-knit bond forged by those sharing the responsibility of caregiving. One of the first things they discuss is what is in it for the caregivers. What are the caregivers' fears about caregiving and what are the benefits they expect to receive? You wouldn't expect benefits from caregiving for someone who is slowing leaving you, but the benefits are real.

According to Sheila Warnock, co-author of the book, in the section of her book, *The Special Benefits of Being Part of a Caregiver Group*:

"As people played their unique roles in caring for someone else, their priorities seemed to shift from reasoning to trusting, from revering the intellect to revering the mystery, from looking good to doing good, from living in the future or the past to living in the moment, and from accomplishment to meaning.

Some people said they felt more connected to humanity. Some said they began to see how we all share the same fears, needs, and desires. Other felt they got a sense of their own place in the world—a sense of belonging. They found out more about their own strengths and weaknesses and they began to acknowledge the strengths and accept the weaknesses. They realized that having limits doesn't mean you're bad or weak, or that the job won't get done."

If you would like to know more about the program visit their website at www.sharethecare.org.

Has your loved one already decided who will have Durable Power of Attorney (POA), Durable Healthcare Power of Attorney, who will handle their finances, how to pay for their long-term care and final arrangement? What about the driving discussion?

At what point will you no longer be able to take care of your loved one? When is a dementia care facility appropriate and how will the costs be covered? Insurance, Medicaid, their life savings, or out of your pocket? Does your loved one have assets that can be sold to pay for care? Will other family members object?

What about potential for elder abuse—financial or physical?

What about other chronic illnesses?

Many caregivers experience burn-out, depression, anxiety, and hypertension, due to the emotional and physical demands placed on them from caregiving responsibilities. What about respite care for you when you are getting close to a tipping point?

There is no such thing as a perfect caregiver but planning ahead or at least being aware of what is coming can make the difference between guilt-ridden burnout and good memories.

> **Elder Abuse** is a single or repeated act or lack of appropriate action, occurring in any relationship where there is an expectation of trust, which causes harm or distress to an older person.

One thing to consider, space is usually available for private pay patients such as those with long-term care insurance, but space is often limited for those on public support. You may have to wait up to a year or more for space to become available.

Cost of Care Rule of Thumb

Whatever you think the cost of care will be, even if it is taking care of your loved one in your home or theirs, multiply it by 3 times to get closer to the actual cost. Depending on where you live the monthly cost to care for someone with dementia or Alzheimer's Disease can range from $1,500 to $12,000 per month. Medicare estimates they pay more than $275,000 per year to care for a person with Alzheimer's Disease in a skilled nursing facility.

The common costs of in-home care include:

- Ongoing medical treatment for dementia or Alzheimer's-related symptoms, diagnosis, and follow-up visits
- Treatment or medical equipment for other medical conditions
- Safety-related expenses, for example home safety modifications or safety services/tracking devices for a person who might wander
- Prescription drugs
- Personal care supplies, for example incontinence supplies or adult wipes

Other options to consider are adult day care, visiting nursing services, in-home care and/or full-time residential care services.

The ability of your loved one to pay for care is one of the main reasons why family caregivers donate so much of their time every year to unpaid family care. When you consider the added burden of food, housing, car maintenance, and added taxes to the equation, it might not be less expensive than assisted living.

Most of us don't know our loved one's financial situation. Let's say you are taking care of a parent. Do you have Durable Financial Power of Attorney, so you can access their bank accounts, insurance policies, pension, or other assets for the arrangements toward long term care?

The financial documents you will need to review with your loved one, as soon as the diagnosis is given, if you haven't already done so, are:

- Monthly or outstanding bills
- Social Security payment information
- Pension or other retirement benefit summaries (including VA benefits, if applicable)
- Insurance Policies (including long term care*)
- Deeds, mortgage papers, or other ownership statements
- Bank and brokerage account information — includes checking and savings accounts
- Stock and bond certificates
- Rental income paperwork
- Tax documents
- Letter of Competency. This document is usually created at the time of their will and advanced directives. It is filled out by their long-time physician stating that the person is competent at the time he or she created the legal documents. With the help of an attorney, this document will dispel any ideas that your loved one lacked the mental competency to make their wishes known about medical care, financial and legal decisions, and prevent legal challenges within the family. See chapter *Doctors, Pharmacists and Me, Oh My*, page 53 for more details.
- Access to Safe Deposit Boxes, including keys and permission to access the box

*Long-Term Care Insurance is a special policy that may cover the items not covered by either Medicare or Medicaid.

It might be helpful to figure out which necessary documents are not in place. Which legal documents are needed? This is a good time to consider seeking professional financial and legal advisors for help.

How to pay for care is a difficult decision. Not everyone will have savings, property, or insurance policies to draw from. Help may come from federal programs such as Medicare or state programs, such as Medicaid or low-cost and free community services. Some caregivers may find they must make personal contribution to their loved one's care.

Do they own their own home? Will they be aging in place? If so, a Home Equity Conversion Mortgage (reverse mortgage) is a possibility for a monthly steady income. To qualify for a reverse mortgage the homeowner must be sixty-two years of age or older. If they haven't paid off the mortgage, they must be close to it.

Property is defined as land and anything attached to land. In this case, the property can have a condominium that meets the Housing and Urban Development (HUD) standards or a manufactured home that meets the Federal Housing Administration

(FHA) standards, a single-family home, or a home consisting of one to four units, such as a duplex or triplex.

Be aware there are caveats with a reverse mortgage, which includes that heirs have 30 days to sell the home after the owner passes or it will revert to the lending institution.

If the homeowner is not aging in place, can the property be rented to provide additional income to cover the cost of care? If you have this option available, check with an elder care or estate lawyer to make sure you have the legal authority to manage your loved one's property when he or she is incapable of managing it.

Many adult children, me included, use their own funds to pay for a parent's ongoing care. If you have siblings, where possible, ask them to make an equal contribution. Be sure to consider other people's circumstances. Some may be unemployed or caring for an in-law or have children in college.

If they can't be supportive financially, let them know their time has value. In my own situation for example, my sister took care of the finances while I did the day-to-day care. She would also take our father on outings to give my husband and me a much-needed bit of respite.

When it comes to asking your siblings for contributions, be flexible, and be creative. Don't be afraid to ask for help. If you are not the primary caregiver, *please* offer your assistance and let the primary caregiver know how you can help. Caregiving can be so overwhelming they may not realize they can ask for help or believe they will receive it.

Health Care Directive for Dementia

Dr. Barak Gaster, University of Washington, Seattle, created an advance directive for dementia. It is an Alzheimer's-specific living will that allows you to choose the level of medical care you wish to receive at each stage of Alzheimer's Disease or any other type of dementia. This is a tool to help your family know what to do for you in the event you or your loved ones develop dementia. Once completed, it can be shared with family, trusted friends, and your doctor ahead of you needing it. It should be completed before someone develops dementia.

The Health Directive for Dementia form is a free download for personal use from Dr. Gaster's website: www.dementia-directive.org.

* * *

For additional resources, see Appendix A, page 210.

Chapter 4: Dementia and English as a Second Language

What's Covered in This Chapter

- Where is My Loved One in Her Language Memory?
- When Am I?
- Deaf and Hard of Hearing Community and Dementia

"Whenever I think of the past, it brings back so many memories." ~Steven Wright

We've all enjoyed chatting with our family and friends over the dinner table, debating opinions, settling arguments, sharing memories, and laughter. Over the years we've developed a common bond, through shared inside jokes and shared language. For those with dementia who as an adolescent or adult learned a new language, that new language fades while the dementia propels itself forward, never taking a breath.

Where is My Loved One in Her Language Memory?

Millions of bilingual migrants around the world cope with dementia. If those parents speak only English with their children, whole generations might grow up not speaking their parents' first language.[10] Once dementia affects her second language, speaking skills often fade quickly, leaving her sitting in silence, unable to communicate. As a result, adult children may not know dementia robbed their mom of the means to speak to them. When this happens, agitation increases and her quality-of-life decreases.

The good news is those who have been bilingual since childhood are less likely to lose the use of their second language.[11]

According to David Murphy co-author of *Bilingualism and Dementia: How Some Patients Lose Their Second Language and Rediscover Their First,* "We heard stories from people working in care homes in Ireland, Scotland and Wales that told how bilingual people with advanced forms of dementia and almost no linguistic skills, were transformed by care workers who could speak the patient's mother tongue. As with many people living with dementia, music and song were often the keys that unlocked the flow of words and memories."[12]

Let's take a look through the experience of Myrna Vander Beek. In 1960, when she turned 15, she emigrated from Donegal, Ireland, with her family. She learned English after arriving in the United States. In 1967, she married Johannes Vander Beek, an immigrant from the Netherlands. They agreed they would only speak English with their children because they wanted their children to feel they belonged.

When Johannes died, Myrna was in the early moderate stage of Alzheimer's Disease. She then moved in with her youngest daughter, Anna. The transition into her daughter's home and family life took about six months before Myrna's disruptive behaviors calmed down. A year later, Myrna slipped in the bathtub and broke her hip. She needed more care than Anna could provide, so Myrna agreed to stay at a rehab facility specializing in memory care.

Anna visited her mother every day after work and noticed her mother seemed progressively distant and more confused. However, the nursing facilities' staff assured her they were managing Myrna's pain and that this was normal.

By the end of the second week, Myrna would speak Irish mixed with English whenever Anna talked to her. Anna, not understanding what was happening, slammed her fist on the nightstand next to Myrna's bed. Myrna flinched.

"What is wrong with you? Mom, just tell me what's going on so I can help you," Anna, shaking, shoved her fist into her pocket. "It's not that hard."

By the end of the third week Myrna became withdrawn. She stopped participating in rehab, started refusing to eat, and lay in her bed staring out the window. Whenever Anna spoke to her mother, Myrna stared at her, her eyes glassy. She slowly turned her head back and forth, tears trickling down her face.

The injury worsened Myrna's dementia and her health followed. She declined to the point where she no longer understood English. Frustrated and not feeling well, she did not seem to understand what was going on around her or what anyone was saying to her. Anna, not knowing her mother had lost her second language, could no longer talk to her mother—losing her emotional connection and her temper. If Anna had known her mother had lost her adopted language, she could have sought the help of an interpreter to bridge the gap and re-establish the bond. If she had known music and song could still reach her mother, she could have added music into her visit to maintain their connection and express her love.

If your loved one is hospitalized, it is their right to ask for and get the help of a _free_ translator or 'medical interpreter.' It may not be offered right away; she may need your assistance to get one. For example, Harborview Medical Center, in Seattle, Washington, reported that 'limited English' patients who used this service understood and followed the doctor's orders and were more likely to recover.

With this in mind, a nearby large hospital may be able to help. Many hospitals keep a list of interpreters. For example, Harborview uses interpreters who speak in over 80 different dialects and languages. Take a look at their website https://ethnomed.org/about/interpreter-services/ for ideas of what you might find in your area. Other hospital networks also use Vocational Rehabilitation (VR) interpreters for the hard of hearing and deaf, using, for example, a tablet connected to video services. There can be some challenges with the translations which will improve as the technology improves.

When am I?

Ascertaining where your loved one is on the journey of her decline will help you determine which language she will recognize so you can meet her needs. "When am I?" may sound like a strange question, however, for people with dementia, early childhood memories feel clearer than the loose batch of more recent memories. As the disease progresses, short term memory disappears, and long-term memory lingers. The farther along the great unravel, the farther back in time they travel. At some point they will no longer recognize you or their own reflection in a mirror, but they will recognize earlier photos of themselves. Gauging when in time your loved one thinks they are living, will prolong your ability to stay engaged with them and maintain your bond a little longer.

Putting together memory aids for her in both languages can reduce her agitation, reduce her long silences, reduce her repetitive questions. If younger children are in the home, this can create an activity your children and your loved one can do together.

Pull together photos of her. Start with current photos and include as many as you can, going back to her early life as a child. If you can, increase the photo size so she can see it without glasses. When she seems confused, show her the photos and ask her to pick herself out. Include titles with the photos, such as "This is me at age 2," "This me at age 45," "This is me at age 85." Do not use any photos with more than three people.[13] It will cause greater confusion. Early on, she will recognize all the photos. In later stages you will know *when* she is in her mind so you can figure out how to relate. You can add titles in her first language, if you haven't already done so, so she can still read and understand what she is seeing.

Once you have a feel for *when* she is, especially if it's early in the diagnosis, you can create cueing devices and memory aids in the language she is able to use. Remember, the change from speaking English to her first language happens very fast.[14] If she insists on reading in English, have back-up copies in her first language so you are prepared for a smooth transition and she can remain independent longer. For more information on memory aids see *Memory Aids and The Family*, page 29.

If you do not speak your loved one's first language, you might find help by reaching out to local communities who speak both languages. Check online for communities near you, for example, the Swedish Club, Sons of Italy, Hmong.org. If you are using professional in-home care, check with your provider to see if they offer services in your loved one's first language.

Smart phone apps such as Google Translate can act as a bridge between you and your loved one. You choose the language for the translation, then speak the phrase or question into the phone. The app will then speak the phrase in the chosen language. Be aware that it can get confused by slang and figures of speech. For example, you and your mom are shopping. You found something overpriced. You winked at her, then you said into the app in English for Arabic translation, "That's as high as a cat's back." Your mother would hear, "This is as high as Zahir threw," at which point she might figure it out. Or she might wonder who Zahir is and why did he throw something, then look at you like you're riding the crazy train. The app is not perfect, but it may help bridge the gap and give you both some much needed laughter.

Multilingual resources are available for those who can no longer communicate in English. Both advocacy groups and government websites now contain advice and specific information in languages other than English. A large range of information on dementia is available in languages like Arabic, Spanish, and Chinese, in addition to languages ranging from Armenian to Zomi.[15] See the Resources section for online support under *Translation Languages*, page 223.

Deaf and Hard of Hearing Community and Dementia

Members of the Deaf and Hard of Hearing Community are less likely to be diagnosed with dementia than hearing people.[16] At the time of this writing, not much information on dementia exists for members of the Deaf community.[17] Those with dementia may slowly lose their ability to sign. American Sign Language (ASL) and British Sign Language (BSL), like all signed languages throughout the world, use multi-channel signs. These are complex utterances which combine a mouth pattern and facial expression, a specific gesture located in space and/or on the body and a precise movement. When produced together they give nuanced meaning to what someone is saying using the multi-channel sign.[18] In addition, according to Lindsay Pierce, CODA (Child of a Deaf Adult) and a Marriage and Family Therapist, body language and facial expression are a language we all communicate with. If you as a caregiver sign, "Today, beautiful day!" but you are frowning or your body is slumped with exhaustion, it may communicate something entirely different and not the message you intended.

Interpreter services, including online, are available for the Deaf and Hard of Hearing Community. However, the deaf and hard of hearing may struggle with online or tablet interpreters because of the nuances lost through video, slow connections or other technology issues. In-person interpretation is recommended. In addition to ASL interpreters, Certified Deaf Interpreters (CDI) are also a wonderful resource for the Deaf and Hard of Hearing who have declined in language overall and may need more gestural or pictorial communications. ASL interpreters are limited by their secondary acquisition of the language and the linguistic influences of English on a language that may need to be tailored more gesturally for those struggling with aspects of the signed language overall.[19] What this means is that hearing ASL interpreters are influenced by their understanding of English. Think of it this way, we all learn some level of writing longhand, however, not many of us can write using calligraphy. Those raised in the Deaf community sign using spatial calligraphy. Deaf individuals also tend to have more challenges with English in general, and depending on the skill of the interpreter, it can be another language barrier without a CDI.

The ability to sign, along with body language and spatial movements decline over time making it harder to communicate. Alzheimer's Scotland offers information designed for caregivers of members of the Deaf and Hard of Hearing community, including those with acquired hearing loss, those who are both deaf and blind, and those working with additional physical debilities. They offer a caregiver guide in English in PDF format for free download. See the Resources section for the link to this guide, page 216.

The effort to speak with her in her first language, whether it is sign language or Estonian, may be difficult but is also rewarding. You keep your emotional bond longer, your ability to communicate, your ability to maintain routine and learn a new language in the process.

"The limits of my language means the limits of my world." ~Ludwig Wittgenstein

Chapter 5: To Drive or Not to Drive, that is The Question

"I had to stop driving my car for a while . . . the tires got dizzy." ~Steven Wright

The skill set to safely operate a motor vehicle involves memory, good judgement, the ability to multitask, understand spatial relationships, and physical ability—which includes quick reaction time. At some point, your loved one will no longer be able to drive. The ideal time for the initial driving conversation with your loved one is once the diagnosis is received.

According to the Alzheimer's Association, the following list of warning signs signals when your loved one is no longer able to drive:

- Forgetting how to locate familiar places
- Failing to observe traffic signs
- Making slow or poor decisions in traffic
- Driving at an inappropriate speed
- Becoming angry or confused while driving
- Hitting curbs
- Using poor lane control
- Making errors at intersections
- Confusing the brake and gas pedals
- Returning from a routine drive later than usual
- Forgetting the destination they are driving to, during the trip. This is not the same as being so deep in thought you drive home from work, walk into your home, and realize you meant to go to the grocery store first

When discussing the subject of retiring from driving with your loved one, be sympathetic to his feelings. Remember when you first earned your driver's license? Getting your driver's license was a symbol of independence; losing his is a loss of independence, loss of control, and a powerful reminder that something is wrong.

Take a ride with your loved one. Create a written record of what you have seen him do while driving. Do not confront him during an incident. It will help with the conversation if he is calm. Look for patterns of change over time. Is he relying on a copilot to drive? Is he stopping in traffic for no reason? Does he have trouble navigating a turn, left or right? Are there several minor incidents or a major incident? An isolated issue doesn't warrant alarm, but if there are multiple dents in the vehicle or the garage or mailbox, it will warrant a discussion. You can also share the journal with other family members who might be in denial, and medical professionals when you need documentation for a diagnosis.

When you decide to have the conversation, choose the time of day when he functions best. Ask him to sit down with you and discuss at what point he would like to give up driving even if he hasn't reached that point yet. You can share your record of his driving with him to get the conversation started. If he doesn't want to discuss it, be gentle but honest that there will come a time when he can no longer drive safely. Be sure to emphasize the positive side and offer alternative options. Such as having groceries, meals, and prescription medicines delivered to his home. If he becomes agitated and aggressive, use the distraction technique for aggression (see *Distraction Techniques*, page 99). Do not yell back. You want him to look at you as his advocate, his champion, not his adversary. The Alzheimer's Association put together several videos demonstrating how to have the driving conversation. They are available at alz.org/driving.

This may be the first of many, many conversations surrounding driving. Don't wait to remove the car until he drives into a store front or runs over someone walking down the street.

Encourage him to check with his primary care doctor and pharmacist to make sure there are no issues with medication that might interfere with his driving. Check with his eye doctor to confirm he doesn't need new glasses to maintain his ability to drive. Also check with his Audiologist to make sure he can hear adequately to avoid possible dangers.

When planning ahead, involve his close friends and family so they are familiar with the plan. When you create the plan, include practical safety steps to take:

- Regular driving assessments
- A car Global Positioning System (GPS) monitoring system
- Other transportation options

Keep in mind if he gets lost and wanders, he will no longer be able to navigate public transportation without someone traveling with him.

The next step in the conversation will include a plan for transitioning driving duties to others. Tell him you or another family member will drive him or arrange for his transportation either via a taxi or special transportation service. For information on local resources including special transportation use the Eldercare Locator at www.eldercare.acl.gov. The available options may be limited in small towns and rural areas. Don't hesitate to check with neighbors or church members for help.

Once a driver's license is revoked, the Department of Licensing will issue a state identification card so your loved one still has "ID." Having ID only may not stop him from driving because he won't remember he doesn't have a license.

The Driving Contract

The Alzheimer's Association created a driving contract which allows the person with dementia to assign a trusted person to tell them when they can no longer drive safely and gives permission for the trusted person to take the necessary steps to prevent the person with dementia from driving again. It is available from the Alzheimer's Association at alz.org/driving.

Medical Intervention

If the doctor determines your loved one is no longer safe to drive,[20] ask the doctor to write a letter or prescription stating, "No driving." Presenting him with a letter from an authority (the doctor) will be a reminder that he cannot drive. Have extra copies made in case he tears it up or throws it away. Physicians are also required to report to the Department of Motor Vehicles (DMV) if someone is no longer safe to drive. If the DMV then requests your loved one pass a test, he will have no choice but to take the test.

Make sure you appeal to his sense of responsibility. If he is still resistant, ask him if he would take a driver evaluation from a disinterested third party such as an occupational therapy driving rehabilitation specialist. An occupational therapist can offer advice specific to your loved one's driving goals and need. This should be done every three to six months to evaluate his abilities. To find out if there is a therapist available in your area check the American Occupational Therapy Association's website: https://myaota.aota.org/driver_search/index.aspx.

Other resources are the Automobile Association of America. They offer the Helping Seniors Drive Safer and Longer Program which includes professional driving assessments. For more information visit their website: https://seniordriving.aaa.com/evaluate-your-driving-ability/professional-assessment/, and AARP has their Driver Safety course. Their website is: https://www.aarpdriversafety.org/.

When you have the medical "no driving" conversation, emphasize your love and support for him.

What to do When Your Loved One Becomes Argumentative

When your loved one insists on driving because he doesn't remember he cannot drive anymore, here are a few things you can try to distract him from driving:[21]

- Explain to him that the route changed, or the driving conditions are dangerous and someone else should drive
- Offer to give him a break and drive him so he can enjoy the view
- Arrange for another person to accompany you on the trip who can sit in the back seat and keep him busy. This is important if your loved one is to the stage where he is angry or aggressive
- You control access to the keys. Instead of leaving the keys where your loved one can find them, you keep them. Then scatter five to ten decoy car keys that look like his keys around his living environment. The benefit is he will get extra exercise trying each of set keys
- Tell him he doesn't have insurance right now
- Disable the car so he cannot drive it by removing one of the following:
  o Distributor cap
  o Battery
  o Starter wire
- Have a kill switch installed under the dashboard so the car will not start without the kill switch being thrown. If it is a hybrid (HEV or PHEV) or electric vehicle (EV) use the emergency response cut-off switch to isolate the battery from the electric system
- For cars made after 2000 take out the fuel pump fuse. The gas tank will show there is gas in the car, but he won't be able to start the car because the car's sensor is telling the computer there is no gas
- Suggest to him one of the grandchildren needs a car to run an errand or the grandchild's car broke down and they need transportation until the grandchild gets their car back from the shop. Your loved one will still feel he has ownership of the car. When he asks for the car back, assure him you will call the grandchild to get it back, but you won't get the car back for him. Yet your loved one will still have the hope of getting the car back
- Tell him the car is in the shop waiting for a part that has been recalled
- If it is your spouse, get a new car that he won't be able to figure out how to start

If you choose to disable the car, keep in mind, if the person is a former auto mechanic, they may be able to fix any of the above suggestions until they get far enough into their dementia.

Another option to consider is to sell the car. The money saved from not paying for the insurance, maintenance, or gas may help pay for other forms of transportation. Keep in mind even if they agree to sell the car, they won't remember in two weeks and may accuse you of stealing the car. This will be true even if you didn't sell the car and another family member did.

Silver Alert

If a person with dementia can wander away from home on foot, they can also wander away from home in a car. At the time of this writing, there are 37 states and the District of Columbia with a public notification system for missing persons called a Silver Alert. The Silver Alert broadcasts information about missing persons, usually senior citizens with Alzheimer's Disease or dementia. Several other states have similar systems but use different names and they may have broader coverage which includes children.

The alerts cover a range of media such as radio stations, cable television, and television stations. The alerts usually consist of the person's name, a description of the missing person, their vehicle and license plate number. Silver Alerts can also be broadcast on the variable-message signs on major roadways and can cover neighboring states.

If the person is suspected of being on foot, Silver Alert also uses the Reverse 9-1-1 or other local emergency notification systems. According to the Alzheimer's Association, "Six out of 10 people with Alzheimer's disease will wander from their homes or caregiving facilities. If not found within a 24-hour period, up to half will suffer serious injury or death."

Many wanderers are lost within a 1.5-mile radius of their home, however, there are those who can travel hundreds of miles and think they have only been on the road for thirty minutes. If you suspect your loved one has wandered and you cannot find them close to home, or their car is missing and does not have a GPS tracker, call 9-1-1. For more information on how to handle wandering, see Distraction Techniques, page 110.

* * *

When debating the issue of whether your loved one should continue driving, consider this: is his ability to drive more important than keeping those around him safe? Choose safety over his independence. If you still can't decide, would you want your child or grandchild riding in the car with him driving? Answering that question will tell you what action is needed.

While you are debating, take your car for a spin and let me know if the tires got dizzy.

Chapter 6: Memory Aids and the Family

The most difficult words to hear from a loved one are, "I've got Alzheimer's Disease (A.D.)" or "I've got dementia." Even if you've suspected it for some time, it's still difficult to accept. There are several things you can do for your loved one and for yourself as they walk the path of decline especially in the early stages.

Memory aids, a cueing aid tool, can be a very sensitive topic, especially for someone with A.D. who doesn't want to admit there is anything wrong.

Here are a few ideas to discuss and try with her. Be open to her refusal to use the aids and/or suggestions for alternatives.

In the chapter *Dementia and English as a Second Language*, page 21, under *When Am I*, we discussed the issue of where your loved one is in her personal memory timeline. The goal in creating that memory aid was to find out when in time she thinks she is living. This will help you understand how to help her navigate her shrinking world.[22]

Once you have a feel for *when* she is, especially if it's early in the diagnosis, it is time to create cueing devices and memory aids.

Cueing Devices

Cueing devices are any aid that helps your loved one remember something.

There will come a time when your patience will chunky dunk into the deep end of the pool chased by repetitive questions. You may feel like a screwdriver is being driven into your ear, which I don't recommend, it hurts.

The ability to read is one of the last cognitive functions a person affected by dementia will lose. After life-long practice it becomes an automatic response. This is where cueing devices come in handy.

When she asks, "Where are we going?" consider

Cueing Device Supplies

- 3" x 5" or 4" x 6" Note cards
- White or Canary Colored Notepad
- Black fine point marker

using the following options. In this example, the trip is to the grocery store. Use either a note card or a note pad and write the answer on the paper in large enough print she can read it. Ask her to hold the note for you. When she repeats the question, instead of answering, ask her to read the note aloud. "We are going to the grocery store." This should reduce the number of repetitive questions. Keep the sentences short, no more than eight words.[23]

People with A.D. may lose their sense of touch as the disease progresses. When touching items become a hazard, label the faucets red and blue or put notes near them with the words "hot" and "cold."

Put signs near the stove, toaster, iron, or other items that get hot with words like "Stop" or "Don't Touch—Very Hot!" Make sure the signs are not so close to the heat source that they might catch on fire.

When wandering becomes an issue, put signs on the door like "Closed," "Do Not Enter," or "Stop." (See *Preparing Your Living Environment for Your Loved One*, page 71 for additional strategies.) For more information on how to handle wandering, see Distraction Techniques, page 110.

Helpful tip: If you're using the note pad, take it with you to any doctor's appointments. There will be many times when you will be exhausted and/or overwhelmed. Writing down the instructions will help you remember it better than reading the doctor's after-visit summary and could save you from making a mistake later, and she can read it, too.

Scrapbooks: Memory Devices, Conversation Starters, Keepsakes

In the early-to-moderate stages of dementia, consider creating a scrapbook with and for your loved one. It doesn't have to be fancy, but it does have to be tailored to her daily life and family activities.

For my father, I used a three-ring-binder and assembled photos of daily activities, trips we took on weekends, his friends, places he'd lived, family members—one photo from his youth and one current photo—and lists of his favorite activities. If more than one person was in a photo, I labeled each person in a large font.

> **Scrapbook Supplies**
> - Large Photo album or 3-ring binder
> - 8-1/2 by 11-inch copy paper
> - Plastic page protectors or 3-hole punch
> - Creativity
> - Optional: Tab sheets, scissors, glue, double-stick tape

Do not use photos with more than three people in it. Using photos with more than three people will cause confusion for your loved one when she gets into later stages of dementia.[24] Include what is important to her.

In my father's Memory Book, we included the waxed leaves we picked each fall he lived with us, trips we took, things that made him laugh, and his favorite nursery rhymes.

After trial and error, we learned there should not be more than two photos on a page, and the description of the photo should be very short. Eight words or less. Examples: "My trip to the beach" or "My cat's name is Tiger" or "I love to fish." If it was more than eight words, he would forget the beginning of the sentence before he got to the end.

One of the advantages of the scrapbook is it can be updated regularly to address her changing needs. As the disease progresses, certain pages may be retired or moved to an alternate scrapbook, especially if something on a page upsets her. Or if she doesn't agree with the wording describing the photo, change it to what she wants it to say.

In the later stages of dementia, when she views the scrapbook, it may become a conversation starter about the photo or possibly a brilliant work of fiction. Watch her enjoy the spotlight while you get a breather.

When she is gone, and you've had time to heal, you will have the added benefit of a cherished keepsake.

Cueing Aids and Children

If children are living in the home with a loved one with dementia, make sure they know they are not responsible for Grandpa's behavior issues that are aggressive or negative.

Set some time aside with your children, when you won't be interrupted, to discuss the issues the family is having with the loved one. Discuss favorite activities they used to do with Grandpa and explain why they can't do the activity anymore. Ask your children to figure out activities they can do together with Grandpa they would both enjoy. Examples could be making up adventure stories, or putting together a small puzzle, coloring with crayons. Write them down for future use.

Prior to the activity, review with your children what they intend to do. After the children have spent the time with him, let them tell you about what happened. If the activity did not go as planned because of memory issues, suggest the children help make pages for the loved one's scrapbook, which they can both look at together.

Discuss the cueing aids and memory devices that might help Grandpa. Have them help create the cueing aids and memory devices so they feel involved. Whether it's putting together the memory book or creating flash cards with simple pictures and short sentences. Explain to your children that cards should be one color like white or canary, as multiple colors will cause Grandpa confusion as the disease progresses. Black ink is best for cue cards. A memory book can be colorful, with photos or pictures from magazines illustrating the sentence. Helping create the aids will benefit your children in expressing their feelings, getting to know their own family history, and give them a sense of accomplishment.

For example, once flash cards have been created, as a family, show your children how to use the flash cards with Grandpa based on his body language, gestures, and level of frustration. Make sure your children understand to speak slowly, move slowly; walk don't run—and to ask Grandpa's permission before doing anything. If they don't, Grandpa will defend himself from the perceived attack, which might include hitting them.

It will become easier for everyone involved to identify issues more quickly once your children get to know him better.

Cueing Aids for Questions about Family Members and Friends Who Have Died

Sometimes a loved one will ask about a person who has passed. "Where is my mother?" There are a few ways to handle this. You can tell her the requested person is on a trip, then ask her to tell you about the person and/or look at photo albums of the person.

Here's the don't: for those who want the more direct approach, known as Reality Orientation, you can tell her the requested person is dead. This approach will cause your loved one to relive her grief anew each time. Going through repeated episodes of your loved one's grieving

> **Cueing Aids for Talking About the Deceased**
> - Photo albums
> - Tissue for tears

requires a lot of stamina on your part and is difficult on your loved one. You cannot force her back into "her-old-self," two or more parts of her brain are dying. She can't go there. She is now living an earlier portion of her life. You need to slow down and join her where she is living, whether it's based in reality or not.

Life Beyond Repetitive Questions

Have a conversation with your loved one regarding what they will accept as cueing aids. Part of dementia, especially Alzheimer's Disease, is covering up what she is forgetting, pretending that all is normal. If she feels insulted by the cueing aids, she may throw them away or hide them, so she won't be reminded something is wrong with her. If a particular cueing aid causes a battle, you may want to try an alternate solution.

For example, she may have trouble getting dressed, but still want to do it by herself. She may slam the bedroom door in your face, or she may crumble up the piece of paper that reminds her to get dressed. Ask her if a list of items she might wear will help her. Instead of calling the list "Getting Dressed," call it "Getting Dressed Up."[25] Show a picture of underwear and next to it print "Put on UNDERWEAR"; next show a picture of a shirt or dress and print "Put on SHIRT" (or blouse or dress); next show a picture of socks and print, "Put on SOCKS" (or stockings or nylons); next to a picture of pants, print "Put on PANTS" and when you get to shoes, print "Put on SHOES." Shoes and gloves and shirts with buttons will become more difficult for her as the disease progresses. There will be mistakes, shoes on the wrong feet, gloves on the wrong hands, or clothing that is backwards or inside out. (For help in finding clothing adapted to her needs and current skill level see *Adaptive Clothing* on page 117.)

Be sure to ask if she is comfortable and would like help. If you try to force the correction on her, she will react unfavorably toward you. An ounce of prevention is worth avoiding a black eye.

Plan ahead to a time when she may or may not be able to find something. Perhaps she cannot find the bathroom. Or she doesn't know where to find a glass for water. Print signs for doors and cupboards. For example, "Myrna's Bedroom," or "Bathroom," or "Plates, cups, and bowls." Do not exceed eight words. If you're not sure what size she can see without her glasses, use the following example.

Example:

Size 12

Size 16

Size 20

Size 24

Size 30

Size 36

Size 48

Size 64

Size 72

Ask her to point out which font size she can read without her glasses.

Cueing Aids for Basic Needs

Have some visual aids ready and start with basic needs, such as hunger, thirst, emotional needs, or comfort. For example, a card showing a meal, a glass of water, or a cup of coffee. A pain scale—going from a happy face with zero (0) below it to a sad face with the severity of ten (10) below it, may be helpful. A list of cards with emotions and a face expressing the emotion. Cards that says, "It hurts on my . . ." with photos or drawings or clip art of feet, hands, head, ears, knees, and the like so she can point to it. Clipart or photos on a card of someone hugging a teddy bear may be helpful when all she needs is a hug for emotional support.

During the first night of my father's stay with us, he experienced hypothermia, but couldn't tell us what was wrong. If I had a card showing someone wrapped in a blanket or wearing a coat, we could have saved an ambulance ride to the emergency room.

Very common in women with moderate to later stages of Alzheimer's disease is saying she is taking care of babies, or that something happened to the babies, or we need to be quiet because the babies are sleeping. This is not generally a hallucination. She needs help or quiet because she feels overwhelmed, and the babies were the only words she could remember.

Cue cards could save your sanity.

Cueing Aids for Nighttime

There will come a time when your loved one will wander around the house when you are asleep. This is known as "Sundowners," a condition, which begins in the moderate stages of Alzheimer's Disease, where she will become increasingly confused as evening approaches.

Signs with pictures or clip art may help at this stage to remind her, for example, where to get a cup for a glass of water, or instructions for turning on the TV, or where the bathroom is located. (See *Preparing Your Environment for Your Loved One*, page 71 for additional suggestions.) Make extra copies. When someone with dementia is Sundowning, cueing aids will wander into lands unknown. It may be easier to put up a replacement than to find the missing card.

Remember, nothing is foolproof and losing your cool hurts you both.

Cueing Aids for Hoarding

Hoarding may become an issue farther into the decline. You might notice piles collecting everywhere. For your loved one who hoards, out-of-sight will not be out-of-mind. Once they can't see something, they feel compelled to collect more, whether it's food, junk mail, or aspirin. For someone who is hoarding it is better to overfill their obsession and let them have multiples of an item, so they feel a sense of control.

Consider getting rid of anything with drawers in their living space except perhaps a nightstand. Use open shelving and make sure the shelves are light colored or white. Dark colored shelves or shelves with multiple colors or patterns will cause issues for her as she declines. She will not be able to see as clearly and might miss an object on the shelf that is right in front of her. Alzheimer's Disease, as it progresses, causes tunnel vision, so the items will need to be in her line of sight. For her collections that cause clutter, clear plastic bins are available. It will give her something to rummage through when she is restless or suffering from Sundowners.

> Sundowners is a worsening of behaviors in the evening.

Another option is using the hanging closet organizers, adding a light to the closet helps.

With her help, label each section of the shelves listing the items stored on them. For example: shirts, socks, underwear, mittens, photo albums, button collection. Make sure the print size is large enough for her to read it without glasses. Consider putting an image of the item such as clip art on the label next to the word. There will come a time when she will not recognize words but will recognize pictures.

Having non-perishable snacks available may help reduce the issues with food rotting in a closet, on a windowsill, in a nightstand drawer, in the bathroom, or under the bed. Create a special, highly visible place on a bookshelf in her bedroom where she can store snacks she enjoys, like peanut butter crackers, chips, serving-sized trail mix packets, or cookies. Store them in a clear plastic canister with a sign above it using her first name which says something like, "Myrna's Snacks."

Be prepared for items to wander around your house overnight and her forgetting where she moved it when she wakes up in the morning.

One of my grandmothers thought the FBI broke into the house each night and moved items around. Instead of getting frustrated with her, make it a game every morning finding the missing item and restoring it to its rightful place. The prize for the winner could be a sticker or a favorite snack. "Will work for chocolate."

You may also need to thin her collections while she is sleeping to prevent unhealthy living conditions. If you remove it all you might experience an explosive response. Remember hoarding gives her a feeling of control over her own environment, while dementia robs her of her own sense of control within her environment.

Other things to consider when dealing with hoarding:

- If you thin a collection, remove the trash from the premises immediately. Otherwise she may be dumpster diving to regain her lost possessions
- Cancel magazine and newspaper subscriptions
- Block home shopping channels through her television provider

The Five Magic Words

People with dementia tend to lose nouns first and get stuck on the wrong words because they no longer know the right ones. When your loved one becomes agitated and tells you they're late for work, they may be remembering a time when they worked and need a task, or what they really needed was a drink of water, or they are in pain.

If you explain she no longer works, the temperature in the room might escalate to an argument. Her becoming argumentative probably had nothing to do with you, but it was her way of expressing her frustration because she couldn't get her message across.

Originated by Teepa Snow, try using the five magic words *"Tell me more about that"*[26] when she gets fixated on something. It could be she knows something is wrong but can't get the message through.

If what she says doesn't make sense, for example she might say, "When is the jet landing?" Try asking follow-up questions based on her body language like, "Describe a jet for me," "Show me the jet," or "Show me what the jet does," or "Show me how you use the jet."

Use your cue cards in addition to the questions.

The Five Magic Words and More Phrases
• Tell me more about XXX?
• Describe a/an XXX for me?
• Show me a/an XXX?
• Show me what XXX does?
• Show me how you use XXX?

She can point more easily than she can communicate verbally. The more you practice together, the faster it will be to interpret what she is trying to communicate. Once you've learned how to communicate, teach your family and friends so they can spend quality time with her, and you can get some much needed down time.

Things to Avoid During the Conversation in Later Stages of Dementia

Dementia and A.D. works in much the same way erasing the memory, but A.D. shrinks the brain because two or more parts of the brain are dying.

Once your loved one reaches the moderate stage of dementia, avoid asking lots of specific questions, questions that require short term memory. For example, "Do you remember who this person is?" or "Do you remember where you put your shoes?" or "Why don't you remember we're going to the doctor?"

The "Do you remember" question is the hardest habit to break. It is ingrained in us from early childhood. We bond over shared experiences. We remember. Our loved ones do not remember.

For her, asking the "Do you remember" questions are a form of torture, like stabbing her with a hot poker or stretching her on the rack—holding her accountable for information she no longer possesses.

The same goes for correcting or contradicting something she stated as fact which you know is wrong. For example, while looking at a photo in the photo album of her sister and she says, "Look, my Aunt Bea."

Your gut reaction is to say, "No, that's not your Aunt Bea, that's your sister, Mary."

Why drive up your blood pressure with an argument no one can win? Avoid the corrections, she is happy, and you know you're right. Win-win.

Try saying to her, "Forget remembering, let's make up something."[27] It frees her from having to remember. The rewards are boundless.

The Dry Erase Board Option

If you've ever stayed in or visited someone in the hospital, on the wall opposite the bed is a dry erase board stating the date, who's caring for you, etc.

The dry erase board, also known as the wipe board or white board, is your friend. So are the fun colored, scented markers—only use one color at a time on the board.

At the top: list the day of the week, the month, day, and year. List upcoming activities and doctor's appointments. If you're inclined, draw a picture or write a saying at the

Dry Erase Board Supplies
• 24" x 18" dry erase whiteboard
• Dry-Erase markers
• Dry-Erase eraser

bottom. List things your loved one asks you repeatedly. Do like the hospitals do, hang it on the wall opposite the foot of the bed. After you've updated the board for the day—in letters large enough for her to read them, it's easy to point to it when a frequently asked question comes up. Ask her to read it out loud from the board. This will reduce the number of questions.

Cueing Aids for Medications

In the early stages of dementia, when your loved one is still able to live on her own with assistance, remembering to take medications may be a concern. There are several products available on the market to assist with medication concerns.

Pill minders come in a variety of forms from seven-day pill organizer dispensers to monthly pill dispenser marked for morning, noon, evening, and bedtime. There are prescription bottle caps with talking alarms, sports watches with pill alarms, or talking interactive alarm clocks with 31-day pill organizers.

Check online pharmacies like CVS, Walgreens, or Walmart. In the search field use the term "pill alarms." Confirm with your loved one which might work best for them.

Medications Cueing Aids
• Pill organizers
• Talking bottle caps with alarms
• Sports Watches with pill alarms
• Interactive Alarm Clocks with 31-day pill organizers

Family Members Opposing Cueing Aids

For every family member involved, there will be a strong and varied opinion about what is best for your loved one's care. Some family members will not accept there is anything wrong with your loved one and will fight every decision.

Family Communication Supplies
• Talking stick
• Counselor, Social Worker, or Minister
• Information on Alzheimer's Disease such as from the Alzheimer's Association's website or your loved one's physician

If more than one family member is involved in her care, learn as much as you can about the disease and what to expect as it progresses. Have a family meeting, which includes any children who will be affected. Prior to the meeting make sure everyone knows the current state of your loved one. Set ground rules for the meeting, such as everyone must attend, even if it is via Skype or FaceTime or some other method of virtual attendance, each person gets to speak—uninterrupted—on the subject, and everyone must listen even if they don't like what they are hearing or don't agree.

If you need to, use an aid such as a talking stick, which is passed from family member to family member when it is their turn to speak. If you use the talking stick remind everyone it is not a weapon but a tool to communicate.

If a family member disagrees with the diagnosis, get them some accurate information about dementia. It's surprising how much accurate information will calm the tension in the room.

For families who generally refuse to work together, consider getting outside professional help, for example from a counselor, a social worker, or a minister. They can help keep the family focused on the problems facing them and their loved one and steer them away from old arguments.

Quick Tip: Organize your first meeting in a public place like a restaurant or coffee shop. The public location tends to keep everyone on their best behavior.

Be sure everyone is on board with reminders and other tools, so they do not take away a tool which genuinely helps her function in her daily life. She cannot be forced back into her previous life and behaviors just because a family member or friend is in denial.

Chapter 7: Emergency Preparedness

Natural disasters affect all of us at some point in our lives. Whether losing your home to fire, volcanoes, tornadoes, hurricanes, flooding, or earthquakes, or smaller events like region-wide power outages, loss of the communication systems, or food and water shortages. Then there are the personal earthquakes; perhaps spilling a beverage down your front, having a car accident, losing your job, or other unpredictable event. When someone with dementia goes out of routine, they experience a personal earthquake. Once they are in the moderate stage of dementia, they usually express their feelings through their behavior: fidgeting, agitation, crying, or aggression.

Planning in advance for life's little emergencies, and big ones, will give you some peace of mind. **It's easier to deal with a crisis if you already have a plan in place.**

Someone who has dementia or Alzheimer's Disease (A.D.), even if she acts functional under routine circumstances, won't be able to function as she usually does during an emergency. If you experience a sudden turn in health, like a heart attack, stroke, or illness, where you can't call for help, your loved one might not be able to summon help for you. She might not recognize what the problem is. She could also misinterpret what is happening, preventing you from getting help. For example, keeping emergency medical personnel from entering the premises, because she insists nothing is wrong.

> **What's Covered in This Chapter**
> - Disaster kit
>   - Personal Earthquake Bag for Everything Else
>   - Emergency Car Kit
>   - In the event of an actual emergency
>
> **Quick Tip**: know before you go where the public restrooms are located. Accidents will happen.
>
> - How to Prepare Before You Get Sick or Die
>   - Contingency Starter Plan
>   - One-Time Emergencies
>   - Continuing Crisis Situation
>   - In the Event You Die First

Disaster Kit

The FEMA website Ready.gov encourages everyone to: Build a kit. Make a plan. Practice the plan. Let's look at what you might need in the event of a personal earthquake. Your day will go a whole lot better if you are prepared for most emergencies.

Personal Earthquake Bag for Everything Else

Personal earthquake bags are the adult equivalent of a baby diaper bag merging with the *Ten Essentials of Hiking*. They include spares of everything you may need in the event of an accident— like incontinence, or an incident— like nakedness, or other unexpected events. There will be many. Everyone's needs vary. However, here is a suggested list of items to carry in your loved one's personal earthquake bag:

- A shawl to use as a cover up when naked happens in public places.
- A "busy apron" or fidget quilt designed for Alzheimer's patients or audio book(s) or music
- Spare clothing, including hat, coat, gloves, shoes, shirt, socks, pants and underwear (clothing should be based on your local weather)
- Light incontinence pads or other incontinence supplies, including adult wipes.
- Plastic bags or garbage bags for dirty clothes and garbage
- Toilet paper
- Paper towel
- Copies of emergency medical information including medication list (see *Appendix A* page 210 for an example)
- Carry a copy of her prescription for glasses and spare glasses (if your loved one cannot afford a spare pair, use the glasses from the previous prescription)
- Sunglasses
- Water, Ensure® or similar product, and snacks
- Blanket(s)
- Small pillow for napping
- Small towels
- Comb
- Toothbrush or sponge-tipped swabs with toothpaste
- Toothpaste
- Lip balm
- Lotion
- First aid kit
- Nitrile, latex, or other protective gloves
- Hand sanitizer
- Aloe Vera gel
- Sunscreen
- Antiseptic ointment
- Anti-diarrheal medication
- Flashlight or headlamp
- Batteries
- Multipurpose tool

- Duct tape
- Safety pins
- Sewing repair kit
- Care instructions for family and friends who are giving respite care

You may not need all of the items listed above and you can assemble the items for your bag over time based on her needs.

<u>Emergency Car Kit</u>

Once you've completed the personal earthquake bag for your loved one, it's time to think about your car. According to Ready.gov, the emergency kit for your car should contain these extra items:

- Jumper cables
- Foldup shovel
- Ice scraper
- Car cell phone charger
- Flares or reflective triangles
- Blanket(s)
- Fire extinguisher
- Map
- Kitty litter or sand for tire traction
- Tire chains

<u>In the Event of an Actual Emergency</u>

Natural disasters that cause power outages require a bit more planning when you have a family member with dementia. A confused mind may not recognize the dangers around them. They may not recognize downed power lines or understand the hazards of smoke inhalation. They may panic and become combative during an emergency situation and refuse to budge.

If you've assembled a personal earthquake bag for your loved one, you are well on your way to getting the rest of your emergency needs in place. In the chapter *Preparing Your Living Environment for Your Love One*, night lights are suggested for guiding the way to the bathroom. Using LED nightlights with battery back-up will provide up to 8-hours of low lighting during a power outage. They have a photocell that registers when you turn the lights out, the battery kicks in when the power goes out. Having one installed in all hallways, the bathroom, and bedrooms will make it easier to navigate during short term power outages when you are scrambling to find flashlights.

If you use traditional candles, do not leave your loved one unattended with an open flame. Anything that creates glare or flickering shadows can cause agitation or hallucinations in an already confused mind. Battery powered candles also work as long as they don't flicker.

Preparing in advance for a natural disaster will help you and your family weather the storm. The American Red Cross recommends the following on their website Redcross.org:

1. Assemble an emergency preparedness kit
2. Create a household evacuation plan that includes pets.
3. Stay informed about your community's risk and response plans
4. Use the American Red Cross "Safe and Well" website to alert family members of your status. (Or use Facebook or other social media, if that is how you stay connected)
5. Download the Red Cross "Emergency App" for iPhone or for Android

In order to stay connected with your family outside of the area affected by the natural disaster, keep all of your electronic devices charged. Find out which local business may be able to help you recharge your electronic devices when the power may be down for days. Coffee shops, restaurants, or even local libraries may be able to help if they run on generators. If your loved one is too stressed to cope with staying in a public place while you recharge your devices make arrangements ahead of time to have someone stay with them while you are gone.

There are two types of emergency preparedness kits, one with a three-day supply of non-perishable food and water in a grab and go backpack, and one with a two-week supply of food and water for sheltering in place when weather events or actual earthquakes cut you off from normal service. These items do not have to be purchased all at once. The kit can be assembled over time. A grab and go backpack should be kept under the bed or in a closet so you can grab it quickly if you must evacuate.

Each person will require one gallon of water per day for drinking and sanitation (hand washing, etc.). Additional basic items to include in your kit are:

- Battery-powered or hand crank radio and/or a NOAA weather radio with tone alerts and additional batteries for both
- Can opener if you have canned food in your kit
- Dust mask, to help filter out contaminated air. The dust mask can be used with fires, collapsed buildings from earthquakes or volcanic eruptions
- First Aid kit
- Flashlights with extra batteries
- Food and water for pets
- Garbage bags and plastic ties
- Local maps (cell towers may be damaged, and you may not be able to use GPS)

- Moist towelettes
- Hand sanitizer
- Pliers or wrench to turn off utilities
- Whistle to signal for help

Any perishable items should be checked every six months such as in January and June to make sure nothing has expired. Choose meaningful dates to help you remember.

Additional items to include if you are forced to evacuate:

- Prescription medication and glasses for every member of the family
- Medication charts for every member of the family (see *Appendix A* page 210 for example)
- Infant formula and diapers
- Feminine hygiene supplies
- Personal hygiene supplies
- Liquid chlorine bleach and a medicine dropper. Do not use bleach that has additives like scents, additional cleaners or is color safe. It will make you very ill if you are trying to create safe drinking water
  - Disinfectant: nine-parts water to one-part bleach, example 9 cups water to one cup bleach.
  - Drinking water: One gallon of water to sixteen drops of bleach
- Waterproof, portable container for important family documents such as bank accounts, insurance policies, and identification.
- Cash which includes change and large and small bills
- Sleeping bags or warm blankets for each member of the family
- Complete change of clothing for each member of the family. This should include sturdy shoes, long pants, and long sleeve shirts. If you live in a cool climate, add coats, hats, scarves, and gloves.
- Car cell phone charger or emergency hand-crank cell phone charger (usually combined with a flashlight)
- Matches in a waterproof container
- Fire extinguisher
- Camping kitchen: paper cups, plates, plastic utensils and paper towels
- Paper and pencil or pens
- Non-battery-operated activities for children such as, books, coloring books and crayons or markers, games, puzzles, playing cards

If you want to look at an additional example of a grab and go backpack, go to www.mil.wa.gov/preparedness.

Create an evacuation plan for your family that includes meeting places in your neighborhood and at least one out of town location. Include updates via your favorite social media channel or the Red Cross App. Choose an out-of-state contact person because the local lines may be overwhelmed during an emergency, the long-distance lines will most likely be available for calls. If you have a mobile phone, text messages may get through when phone calls may not. Create a list to include important contact information for doctors, schools, workplaces, or any service providers (such as day care providers or in-home medical assistants).

Make sure every non-dementia family member carries a copy of the evacuation plan with them at all times, in their backpack, purse or wallet. Put the plan in a colored envelope, like lime green, so that you can find it easily when you are digging for it. Label the envelope so everyone knows at a glance what it is without opening it. You can also share an electronic version; however, it may not be available during an emergency if it is not stored on your local device. Access to the Cloud will be cut off until power and communication lines are restored.

Plan family meetings where you review and practice your plan. Include your loved one and any pets. If you rush someone with a confused mind, they will become agitated. Practice the plan in the evenings when she is Sundowning as well as other times of day, so you know what challenges to expect, especially if an emergency occurs at night. Work out the best method for each family member to help her de-escalate if she overreacts. See *Distraction Techniques*, page 99, for ideas.

Adapt your plan based on your practice drills' successes and failures. Make it fun, remember to laugh, include some play time as you develop the plan. Celebrate the successes and the failures. Who is going to be more cooperative if she is having fun? Your loved one, that's who.

Practice and preparation will streamline your ability to evacuate safely. The more you run practice drills, the calmer every member of the family will be in the event of an emergency, including your pets. It's easier for everyone to rely on a familiar routine. Routine reduces mistakes. The key to successful dementia care is routine. If you keep the drills light-hearted, she will be more cooperative, and you may have some great memories after she passes. The best memories are created in the small moments. *"Remember the time . . ."*

During a disaster, your neighbors are the most immediate source of help. Many local emergency operations centers offer a course called *Map Your Neighborhood*. It focuses on one street at a time. Basically 15 to 20 homes or an area you can walk around in one hour. The course covers the steps to take following a disaster when emergency services are not available for the first few hours, days or even weeks. It teaches how to organize your neighbors and know who has what skills and supplies that may be useful in a disaster. The course teaches how to create a neighborhood map showing the locations of propane tanks and natural gas lines in your neighborhood and how to work together as a neighborhood.

How to Prepare Before You Get Sick or Die

The only two things in life said to be certain are death and taxes. We aren't here to worry about the taxes. Life is full of the unexpected. Whether it is the need for surgery or passing suddenly, when you are caring for someone with dementia, you need to have a back-up plan in place.

Contingency Starter Plan

Let's start with a contingency plan should you become ill or break a bone or need surgery. This is a one-page sheet you will fill out and give to family, friends, hired caregivers, your supervisor at work and co-workers prior to any emergency.

At the top of the page you will include your name and contact information and the name of your loved one. At the bottom of the sheet include the date it was created or updated. It will be updated when life changes happen for the contacts on your list. They may change jobs or move, or some other life event may prevent them from helping you.

Include in the list the names and phone numbers of:

- Those who can provide substitute care for your loved one while you are incapacitated
- Those who can provide alternate transportation for your loved one
- Those who can substitute for you at work. Check with your supervisor or manager to make sure they agree with your choice(s).

Consider you may need a back-up plan for the adult and/or child daycare center, your children's school(s) or even your home. Try to think of any crisis scenarios that could happen with each of these places and give a copy in a brightly colored envelope to someone you trust at each location. Label the envelope so everyone knows at a glance what it is without opening it. Creating this plan and sharing it will help everyone involved know what to do and who to contact in the event of an emergency. It will give you some peace of mind.

One-Time Emergencies

There is always the possibility an unexpected event will occur preventing you from returning home in a timely manner. In my case it was a double fatality on the only bridge servicing our small town. Gridlock kept me on the road for eight hours one evening and I nearly ran out of gas. Stuff happens.

Write out your loved one's schedule in a routine list and ask a trusted family member, friend, or even a hired caregiver if she would be willing to be your emergency back-up to pick-up your loved one from an adult daycare center and/or stay with your loved one until you reach home. Make sure they have a way to access your home if necessary.

Include the following on her daily routine list:

- The time she gets up from bed and morning routine
- What she eats and drinks for breakfast
- Toileting schedule
- What medications she takes:
    o When she takes them
    o How she takes them
    o Where they are stored
- Attach the list you created for the Emergency Medical Technicians (EMT's). See *Doctors, Pharmacists, and Me, Oh My*, page 53.
- Your loved one's daily activities including art projects, hobbies, napping, and exercise
- What time they eat lunch and favorite foods
- Any afternoon activities and suggestions for coping with Sundowning. Include a copy of her Meltdown Trigger List so they know how to avoid a trigger leading to a meltdown. (See *Distraction Techniques*, page 102)
- What time they eat dinner and their favorite foods
- What is their routine after dinner?
- What time do they go to bed, what do they wear to bed and what grooming do they do before they go to bed. Example: wears plaid pajamas, brown wool gloves, and pink bunny slippers, and needs help brushing teeth, toileting, and combing hair, sleeps with her stuffed-toy, baby seal named Alexander
- If your loved one wanders the halls at night, include that on the schedule
- List any actions on the caregiver's part that may cause agitation or aggression in your loved one and how to avoid it or deescalate it

The more your back-up knows, the better the outcome for everyone involved.

Continuing Crisis Situation

Should you become incapacitated for a longer period, such as recovering from a heart attack, stroke, broken bone, or surgery, you will need to make longer term arrangements for your loved one's care.

Here are some things to consider when you are planning:

- Arrange for someone who can relieve you from caregiving for the time you will be down such as a sibling, spouse, a member of your church, or a professional caregiver. Give him or her a copy of your loved one's routine and the duties that need to be done

- Locate suitable paid respite care options. Check with your local Area Agency on Aging for recommendations on care facilities. For local listings, check with the Association of Area Agencies on Aging: www.n4a.org. Once you've identified a care facility you would like to use, confirm how much advanced notice they need to accept your loved one. Most facilities can accommodate requests when given 24 hours' notice
  - If you use this facility regularly to ensure you get regular down time, your loved one will already be familiar with the facility and have fewer issues with any transitions

Once you have this in place, your loved one's routine will be intact, and you will be able to recover.

You will need the following documents for yourself in the event you need long-term care:

- Durable Financial Power of Attorney (this can be covered under Durable Power of Attorney)—allows someone you choose to manage your finances in the event you are unable to make the decisions for yourself, due to something like an illness or dementia. It grants the person you choose to act for you in your financial affairs. The official title of the person you name varies by state, but they are often referred to as your agent or attorney-in-fact

- Durable Power of Attorney, Health Care—a document in which you appoint someone to be your representative or agent in the event you are unable to make your wishes known. Your representative will make the decisions about all the aspects of your health care

If the person you appoint as your durable financial power of attorney is not the same person as your durable medical power of attorney, there is a potential for conflict.

If they disagree on your medical care, the financial agent can make your getting medical care very difficult.

In the Event You Die First

The last item, and perhaps the most difficult emotionally, is arranging for permanent care in a skilled nursing facility for your loved one in case you die or become terminally ill. While it is unlikely that you will precede her in death, making a written plan called a *Letter of Instructions* is vital so those left behind will know what to do.

Here are some things to consider when you are planning:

- Is there long-term care insurance, or Medicaid available to pay for the cost of care? Write it in your plan
- If the facility is private pay (covered by long-term care insurance) are you pre-registered?
- For many facilities covered by Medicaid, you will need to get on a waiting list more than a year in advance to ensure space is available

Create a Survivor's Binder that includes the following information:
The legal documents you will need to have in place:

- Letter of instructions — make this the first page of your binder
- Funeral or burial arrangements and instructions, including if you elect to donate your organs or donate your body to science
- Your will — this legal document tells who will manage your estate, who will get your belongings, and, if applicable, who will become guardian of your minor children or other disabled family members after you die. If you die without a will, the state makes these decisions — often at an added cost to those you love most
- Your Digital Estate — this is a document that lists all of the websites you visit regularly, such as banking, insurance, or online bill pay, social media, email, video and music streaming sites. Include your

> A *Letter of Instructions* is an informal document that gives your survivors information concerning important financial and personal matters that must be attended to after your demise. You don't need an attorney to prepare it. Although it doesn't carry the legal weight of a will and is in no way a substitute for a will, a letter of instructions clarifies any special requests to be carried out upon death. It also provides essential financial information, thus relieving the family of needless worry and speculation. Just as with all your other estate planning documents, be sure your loved ones know where your letter of instructions is located.

usernames, security challenge information, and passwords. Like the letter of instructions, it is not a legal document and should not be included in your will. Your will is a public document and is released to the public upon your passing during probate. Instead, specify in your will where you keep the document. For more information on digital estates and how to close down social platforms see *Digital Estates and How to Deactivate a Loved One's Social Media, Email Accounts, and Other Digital Estates*, page 196

- <u>Durable power of attorney</u> — delegates the power to legally handle your financial affairs should you become disabled or incapacitated. Without this, no one may be able to access your bank account, securities, or any other property in your name without lengthy legal proceedings. Powers of attorney end with your death

- <u>Advanced Directive</u> — a catch-all term that refers to health care directives, living wills, health care (medical) powers of attorney, and other personalized directives. All of these documents allow you to express legally your preference for continued health care should you become terminally ill. A health care power of attorney (also called a "designation of health care surrogate") names a spouse or trusted relative to make health care decisions for you in case you are physically or mentally incapable of doing so on your own

- <u>Letter of Competency</u> — this document is usually created at the time of your will and advanced directives. It is filled out by your primary care physician stating that you are competent at the time the legal documents were created. With the help of an attorney, this document will dispel any ideas that you lacked the mental competency to make your wishes known about medical care, financial and legal decisions, and prevent legal challenges within the family. See chapter *Doctors, Pharmacists and Me, Oh My*, page 53 for more details

Note: If the deceased person had a Durable Power of Attorney for Health Care Decisions (DPAHC) or an Advance Health Care Directive (AHCD), the person they named as their agent is the one who has the legal right and responsibility to arrange for the disposition of the remains (burial, cremation, or donation) per your instructions.

The financial documents you will need to have in place are:

- Monthly or outstanding bills (this can be listed in a spreadsheet). Be sure to include:
  - The company's name
  - Account numbers
  - Company contact information

- o Any security information required to prove your survivor is your heir or executor
- Social Security income information (if you are eligible). This will require your social security number and personal information
- Pension or other retirement benefit summaries (including VA or railroad benefits, if applicable)
- Insurance policies
- Deeds, mortgage papers, or other ownership statement
- Bank and brokerage account information—includes checking and savings accounts
- Safety deposit box information (have your designated heir or executor included on the signature card)
- Stock and bond certificates
- Rental income paperwork
- Tax documents

Medical and other documents you will need for your loved one's continuing care:

- Medication list
- Medical history including:
  - o Allergies to medications
  - o Past surgeries
  - o Ongoing health issues (for example: diabetes, gout, arthritis, sexually transmitted diseases, heart disease, stroke, cancer, kidney failure, smoking, drinking alcohol, GERD—also known as acid reflux, benign prostatic hyperplasia, also known as an enlarged prostate, impotence, immunocompromised—meaning they can't fight infection or other diseases, etc.)
  - o Family history, including what deceased family members died from
- Meltdown Trigger list, if you created one
- Daily Routine list

It is okay to do a little bit at a time. If you feel like you are in over your head, ask for help. If you need the help of a professional, ask for their rates and the amount of time needed to prepare the documents ahead of engaging their services. If you feel like you are being pressured into something you don't understand and they are not explaining it clearly, it's okay to walk away and chose another professional.

Another excellent resource available for free is AARP's Prepare To Care guide, accessible online at:

https://www.aarp.org/content/dam/aarp/home-and-family/caregiving/2012-10/PrepareToCare-Guide-FINAL.pdf . There is an in-depth section at the end of the guide which includes a place to list legal, financial, and medical contacts with spaces for medications, Medicare information, VA Benefits, which bills are due and when, passwords, and a host of other things you will need to know to prepare for that next step.

Once this information is in one place, make sure a trusted family member or friend knows where to find your binder or documents.

Emergencies are never easy but having the resources in place to cope with whatever you may face will lower your stress levels. Remember the importance of self-care. You are worth the effort. Be prepared.

Chapter 8: Doctors, Pharmacists, and Me, Oh My

If you take care of the small things, the big things take care of themselves. ~ Emily Dickinson

Setting the Records Straight

Keeping good medical records will give you peace of mind and cover any of your own memory lapses when you are too tired or overwhelmed to remember everything. You won't remember everything—even if you have an elephantine memory, some little details will slip through. You might not remember every one of your loved one's surgeries, like when your mom had her funny bone surgically removed in 1999 after you drove her new car into the mailbox waving at the cute boy next door. It was so last century.

Over the course of her care, there will be a lot of medical documents you need to keep track of.

It doesn't have to be fancy, just a file box and some manila file folders to label. Give each file a specific name. For example, "Medications" or perhaps "Prescriptions," "Medicare Documents," "Supplemental Insurance," "Hospital Bills," "Doctors," "Documents for Doctors Appointments," "Legal Documents" and any other additional files you may need. You will be surprised how much time it can save you not having to dig through piles trying to find what you need at the last minute. You can also keep an e-file on a thumb drive for back-up.

It may not seem important now, but if she is seeing multiple doctors, being able to pull together all the pieces of paper may prevent other doctors from prescribing medications with an unintended side effect.

Keeping track of all of her doctors, where they are located, upcoming appointments or surgeries can also be overwhelming. See *Appendix A*, page 210, for a sample spreadsheet for tracking doctors' appointments, addresses, phone numbers and other important information.

What's Covered in This Chapter
- Setting the Records Straight
- Doctors' Appointments
  - Advanced Care Planning
  - Testing for Other Illnesses
  - Healthcare Power of Attorney
  - Letter of Competency
  - POLST Explained
- Your Pharmacist is Your Friend
- Signs and Symptoms of Common Health Issues
  - Urinary Tract Infections
  - Hearing Loss and Dementia
  - Hypothermia
  - Stroke
  - Heart Attack
  - Working with Emergency Medical Services
  - The Personal Earthquake Bag Revisited

Doctors' Appointments

The first time you take your loved one to a primary care physician's (PCP) appointment or any other doctor's appointment, if this is a new physician, make sure your loved one is comfortable with the provider's gender. For a first appointment you will need her insurance information, a copy of her medical history, a list of current medications, a copy of your health care power of attorney, a list of concerns you want to cover during the visit, a pad of paper and pen for notes (see *Memory Aids and the Family*, page 29) and a log of any noticeable changes in behavior (See *Distraction Techniques*, Meltdown Trigger List, page 102). If this is a physician she is established with, you need to bring insurance information, any changes in her medical history and changes in her medication list.

Always bring *copies*, not the original, of the legal forms and medical histories for visits because you may not get them back. If you lose the original, it will be very difficult to replace. If arranging for copies is difficult, ask the physician's staff to make copies of the documents for you. As more medical practices go paperless, they may scan your information and return the documents to you.

Medical history includes dates of surgeries and significant events; ailments, such as arthritis, eczema, COPD, or heart disease; what deceased family members died from; allergies; and life style choices like exercise, sex, smoking, alcohol and use of recreational drugs. Include in the history if your loved one is a member of the LGBTQIA+ community. This is important for their providers to know about as a lifestyle choice, so the provider does not overlook important care needs, which might not otherwise be addressed. (See SAGEUSA for more information on the LGBTQIA+ community in *Resources* page 227.)

> **Copies of Paperwork for Doctor's Appointments**
> - Medicare Card (if applicable)
> - Medical Insurance Card and Supplemental Insurance cards
> - Medical History
> - List of Medications
> - Health Care Power of Attorney
> - List of any concerns, such as symptoms, to cover for visit
> - Pad of paper and pen

It's important to know what medications, including all supplements and vitamins, she is taking, who prescribed it, and what each one is used for. In *Appendix A*, page 210, there is an example form listing medications, dosage, instructions, use, and prescribing doctor. It also includes her name, her date of birth, her primary care physician's name and the date it was last updated.

During the doctor's appointment, use the notepad and pen. There will be many times when you will be exhausted and/or overwhelmed. Writing down the instructions will help you remember them better than reading the doctor's after-visit summary, and could save you from making a mistake later.

When she progresses further in her dementia and she becomes argumentative over the instructions, have her sign the physician-provided after-visit summary at the doctor's office and the doctor initial it or sign it. It gives you written proof and may help her when she cannot even remember visiting the doctor. People who are unable to think clearly will respond more cooperatively if they believe it is coming from a person of authority. Forms provide authority for those with confused minds. If she becomes argumentative about signing the form, smile or groan with empathy and tell her it is a requirement of the insurance company. You will get a lot of mileage playing the "insurance company" card, and you won't be the villain.

During the appointment concerning dementia, the staff will perform a memory test. It might be the Montreal Cognitive Assessment (MoCA) or, as in the following examples, a Mini-Mental State Exam (MMSE). She will be asked questions like "Where are you?" "Can you count backwards from 100 by 7's?" "What season is it?" "What day of the week?" "Who is the president?" "Can you spell 'world' backwards?" "When is your birthday?" Each question is designed to assess her mental state and measure any decline. It is an assessment tool, not a diagnosis. Further testing must be performed to eliminate other health issues and confirm a dementia diagnosis. Please note, Medicare covers the cost of the cognitive exam under the annual wellness visit.

A survey of American physicians by the Alzheimer's Association in 2019 noted that less than 50% of doctors even broach the subject of memory issues with their senior patients during a visit,[28] so if you notice sudden changes, bring this to the attention of your loved one's care provider sooner rather than later, so an assessment can be done.

Advanced Care Planning

During your initial visit with her doctor, it is a good time to start the process of advance care planning. When she is in the early stages of dementia, she should be as involved as possible in her own planning.

Not all doctors are comfortable with advance care planning. If this is the case, be sure to ask the doctor to review her overall medical status and what conditions are most likely to affect her beyond the dementia. Check with her doctor to find out what health concerns you might expect over the next year or two.

During the appointment, ask the doctor to direct questions to your loved one. It is too easy to talk around someone with dementia as though they are not in the room, but it only adds to their frustration and feelings of helplessness over losing their sense of self.

If the doctor directs questions to you instead of your loved one, be polite, but say, for example, "This is my mom's appointment, please ask her. I'll help when she needs me to."

Don't be afraid to ask the doctor if there is a way to simplify a care plan to make it more doable. Most doctors can do this for you, but you have to request it. It can be difficult for a loved one with insulin-dependent diabetes or other chronic illnesses to manage things like "as-needed medications." Other examples would include asthma, pain, or Chronic Obstructive Pulmonary Disease (COPD).

If you notice a sudden downturn in her dementia also known as delirium, ask her doctor to check for other chronic illnesses. Most older adults experience more issues than just dementia. It could be she has a bladder infection, untreated pain, constipation, or side effects from medication. Taking care of an issue once you notice it can save a trip to the emergency room, which will create its own complication for her and the emergency personnel who are trying to help.

<u>Testing for Other Illnesses</u>

If it is a more serious issue, such as cancer, and the doctor wants to take a biopsy (sample of affected tissue), consider how the procedure and treatment will affect her. Has she been hospitalized repeatedly over the past few years due to something like congestive heart failure or kidney failure? What are the pros and cons of treatment? She may not understand what is happening to her and may not be able to handle the stress the treatment places on her.

Ask the following questions of her doctor:[29]

- Is the treatment likely to be stressful for her?
- What will happen if we just watch it? "It" being whatever the condition is.
- It may turn out that full treatment is not necessary based on her current conditions. If a major treatment is decided upon, ask the following:
    - How will this help with her overall care?
    - What are the possible stressors she will experience?
    - Would sedatives or anesthesia use be hard on her?*

*Anesthesia can cause, or worsen, dementia in older adults. It is known as post-operative cognitive decline (POCD) and is thought to be associated with inflammation in the brain, similar to what is seen in Alzheimer's Disease.[30] Younger adults without cognitive decline tend to bounce back from the affects after surgery.

Most doctors focus on the treatments and procedures and do not focus on how it will affect someone with dementia. Be very specific when asking how the test results may help better manage her overall health. Focus the doctor's attention on the big picture. It can be very difficult for specialists to focus outside of their branch of medicine.

Will she defend herself during the treatment because she no longer understands what is going on? For example, if she no longer remembers she has failing kidneys, will she understand why someone is trying to stab her with a needle for dialysis? Will she feel threatened and punch the medical provider who is trying to help her?

You need to know what issues you must focus on at her present stage of dementia.

Quick Tips for doctor's appointments:

- Arrive early allowing for time to use the restroom prior to the appointment
- Bring water, a snack, and any medications your loved one might need in case the appointment is delayed
- If fidgeting or restlessness is an issue, bring along an activity for your loved one like a fidget quilt or soft book to keep her occupied

Healthcare Power of Attorney

Durable Power of Attorney Health Care (Health Care POA) is a document which lets her choose a trusted person to make health care decisions for her when she can no longer make those decisions for herself.

It includes such issues as:

- What medical care she receives
- Medications
- Surgeries
- Medical diagnostic tests
- Moving into a long-term care facility or assisted living facility
- Life sustaining treatment and resuscitation

When your loved one passes, if she had a Durable Power of Attorney for Health Care decisions (DPAHC) or an Advance Health Care Directive (AHCD), the person she named as her agent is the one who has the legal right and responsibility to arrange for the disposition of her remains.

All other powers of attorney end with her passing.

Letter of Competency

This document is usually created at the time a person's will and advanced directives are documented, or when updates need to be made. It is especially important if the person has mild memory loss. It is filled out by the person's long-time primary care physician stating that the person is competent at the time he or she created the legal documents.

In some cases, it may be necessary to obtain this letter from a psychiatrist or neurologist who specializes in mental health and cognition. With the help of an attorney, this document will dispel any ideas that your loved one lacked the mental competency to make their wishes known about medical care, or financial and legal decisions and prevent legal challenges within the family.

Creating additional proof of mental capacity when changing or creating any legal document may feel excessive, but you never know whether a family member or stepparent may challenge the validity of legal documents. This could lead to lengthy court battles over wills or guardianship or even an investigation by Adult Protective Services (APS).

The following should be included in a letter of competency:

- Patient's name
- Patient's date of birth
- The original date the patient-physician relationship was established
- Physician's statement attesting to the patient's ability or inability to make decisions, independent of others, regarding their healthcare, finances, and legal matters
- The patient's medical diagnoses, such as Alzheimer's Disease, developmental delay, mental illness, or stroke
- Date of diagnosis for any medical issue relevant to competency
- Physician's contact information

The letter should be printed on the physician's letterhead.

Work with your attorney to determine if any other supporting evidence should be included in the letter. File the original letter of competency with the other corresponding legal documents in a safe place.

POLST Explained

The Physician's Orders for Life Sustaining Treatment (POLST) is an important document that will communicate your loved one's wishes if she is found unconscious. It covers several topics.

Section A of the POLST allows her to choose under what circumstance can someone perform Cardiopulmonary Resuscitation (CPR) if she has no pulse and is not breathing.

Something to consider with CPR and aging is the older a person gets, the more brittle the bones become. At what point does it become cruel to break someone's bones to keep them alive a little longer? Will she contract pneumonia because of the broken bones if she survives?

Section B covers *Medical Interventions*, meaning the person has a pulse and/or is breathing.

> *Oral Suction* uses a rigid plastic tube called a Yankauer to remove excess fluids from the back of the mouth and top of the throat at the pharynx.

- Does she want comfort measures only such as oxygen, oral suction, and manual treatment of airway obstructions, wound care, or other measures to relieve pain and suffering, but does not want to be transferred to a hospital?
- Does she want *Limited Additional Interventions* which in addition to the above include medical treatment, includes IV fluids, cardiac monitoring but no use of intubation or mechanical ventilation (breathing)? This includes transfer to a hospital but avoids intensive care
- Does she want *Full Treatment* which includes all of the above plus the use of intubation, advanced airway interventions, mechanical ventilation and cardioversion? This choice includes transfer to the hospital and includes intensive care

> Cardioversion is a treatment for an irregular heartbeat, also called arrhythmia, atrial fibrillation or AFib. It sends electric shocks through electrodes attached to the chest to the heart, restoring it to a normal beat.

Section C covers the use of antibiotic and what level of use would be preferred between none to prolonging life if possible.

Section D is artificially administered nutrition. This is the section which discusses tube feeding to prolong life.

Section E includes medical conditions and overall goals for the patient.

Section F are the signatures of one of the following: the doctor, Advanced Registered Nurse Practitioner (ARNP) or Physician Assistant-Certified (PA-C), their phone number, date they signed and the patients or legal surrogate's signature. The POLST is usually displayed above the patient's bed and available for emergency medical personnel.

The POLST also supplies optional additional contact information and lets other medical professionals know if there is a Health Care Directive (Living will), Durable Power of Attorney—Health Care (DPOAHC) or a living will registry. The last section contains directions for health care professionals using the POLST.

Keep in mind not all medical staff will be fully versed in the instructions contained in the POLST. They may withhold treatment assuming that is the intended use of the document if they are caring for someone with a POLST. If your loved one is not conscious to confirm she wants treatment and you are the Medical POA, you are her advocate.

This form should be reviewed periodically and updated as her conditions change. She may initially want to be resuscitated but may change her mind as her health declines. Choose a special day that you will remember like Valentine's Day or the first day of spring. Then once you have updated the document, you can celebrate the day together. Do I hear chocolate bunny ears in your future?

Your Pharmacist is Your Friend

One of the most overwhelming responsibilities when first caring for a loved one is getting a handle on their medications, dosages, whether the medication should be taken with or without food, and medication timing. When she is in the early stages of dementia or A.D., she may only need prompting to remember to take her medications. Even simple tools like talking clocks or alarmed medication caps can help retain independence longer (See *Memory Aids and the Family* page 38 for more prompting devices.) If she has trouble swallowing, ask your pharmacist if a liquid version is available or if the medication may be crushed and mixed with food or drink.

However, if your loved one is seeing multiple doctors, it might be a good idea to visit your pharmacist and request a drug interaction check. Your loved one's doctor may not know all of the interactions between medications.

Once you have the results back from the pharmacist, create a list of the medications, their dose (strength), directions for use, and the reason for the medication. Review this with her doctor along with the notes from the pharmacist, especially if there are any adverse drug interactions.

Once the medication list is updated, keep a copy for each doctor's visit and for emergency medical personnel in the event of an emergency. Be sure to include your loved one's name and date of birth to prevent any mistakes on the part of Emergency Medical Services (EMS) personnel or hospital staff.

An example from my own life: When we brought my father home, we were able to remove 22 drugs prescribed by several different physicians who had no knowledge of the adverse drug interactions the medications may have caused. Based on the drug interaction report provided by the pharmacist, the removal of those medications reduced his dementia from borderline severe to early moderate. It did not stop the dementia; it gave him three more quality years. Results will vary depending on the person and the drug interactions.

See *Appendix A*, page 210, for a sample Medication Chart.

Signs and Symptoms of Common Health Issues

There may be times when your loved one has a non-dementia related health issue but doesn't have the capacity to tell you. Very few of us have medical or first aid training. Knowing the signs to watch for may help you get the right medical attention for her needs or prevent a trip to the emergency room. When in doubt, call 9-1-1.

<u>Urinary Tract Infections</u>

Be prepared for "inappropriate toileting," when a loved one will not remember what a toilet is and will use something else in her confusion. This is different from incontinence when they may have an accident in their clothing. Incontinence may be caused by certain medications like diuretics or a urinary tract infection (UTI). It can happen at any time.

Watch for the following UTI symptoms:

- An urge to urinate (pee) that can't be delayed
- Burning or pain when urinating
- Very little urine
- Urine tinged with blood
- Complaints about soreness or pain in their sides, back, or lower abdomen
- Signs of nausea, vomiting, chills, or fever, when an infection hasn't been caught in the early stages

After a UTI has been ruled out and your loved one has not yet transitioned to adult diapers, here are some ideas to help prevent accidents.

For one thing, our bodies have natural times when we use the bathroom. So schedule toileting every two to four hours. A cued trip to the toilet may reduce the frequency of accidents or eliminate them entirely.

If your loved one refuses to give up her chosen spot for toileting, typically overnight or during sundowners, try lining the chosen area with incontinence pads or dog training potty pads from the local pet store. If you prefer something machine washable with odor control built in, try Pooch Pads from poochpad.com. In some cases, they may be less expensive than the pharmacy supplied incontinence pads. Remember, nothing is foolproof.

Be sure to have a conversation early on with your loved one about when they would be willing to wear absorbent products for incontinence (adult diapers). Who knows, someday we may even order them from Victoria's Secret.

Hearing Loss and Dementia

There is a strong correlation between hearing loss and dementia.[31] This doesn't mean that people with hearing loss are guaranteed to get dementia, it just means the odds are higher. If someone experiences hearing loss, their brain must work harder to interpret the sounds it does hear, which may take away resources that their brain would use for other important functions. Additionally, if their ears no longer hear as many sounds, the hearing nerves will send fewer signals to the brain causing further decline.

Many of the symptoms of hearing loss are similar to those of Alzheimer's disease. Hearing loss is known to affect speech and speaking skills. There is also a common link to depression with both hearing loss and dementia.

Using hearing aids may help your loved one stimulate their brain function and increase their willingness to socialize, slowing down cognitive decline. However, not everyone with dementia will want to wear hearing aids. The newly recovered sounds can be overwhelming and frightening. There are also the issues of hearing aids getting misplaced or lost, and your loved one forgetting to replace the batteries.

Hypothermia

Hypothermia can happen for a number of different reasons. If your loved one is stressed, she will become cold. If she has recently moved to an environment that is cooler than her previous living space, she could experience hypothermia. This happened with my father on the first night living with us.

Symptoms of hypothermia can be difficult to recognize in a person with dementia because the first symptom is a change in their mental status such as a change in their personality. You might see aggression, apathy, disorientation, signs of exhaustion, or feeling tired. Is it dementia or hypothermia?

Look for the following symptoms:

- Shivering is usually the first recognizable sign. However, with extreme hypothermia, shivering will stop.
- Fumbling of the hands
- Slurred speech
- Cool stomach. Touch the back of your hand to their skin under their clothing. If your hand is warmer than their stomach, treat for hypothermia.
- Lower core body temperature. This can be very difficult to determine without a digital thermometer which can read below 90°F (32°C).

Someone with mild hypothermia will have a temperature between 90°F (32°C) and 95°F (35°C). Below 90°F (32°C) is severe hypothermia.

If she has hypothermia, get her someplace warm to prevent more heat loss. Treat her gently to prevent cardiac arrest. Replace any wet clothing with dry clothing. Wrap her body with a blanket (electric if available), towel, pillows, sheets, or even newspaper, anything that will prevent further heat loss. Cover her head and neck. If she has mild hypothermia, shivering will help to rewarm her body. Do not give her coffee or alcohol as both will cause her to lose more body heat.

When to Call 9-1-1

If her temperature is below 90°F have her lie down flat while still warming her and call for emergency medical services. She may lose consciousness. If she appears to stop breathing, begin CPR while still warming the rest of her body.[32]

Stroke

People diagnosed with dementia tend to have mixed dementias. According to the National Institute on Aging, mixed dementia is a combination of two or more types of dementia. Any number of combinations is possible, for example a person can have Alzheimer's disease and vascular dementia. It is another reason why no two people with dementia will react or progress the same way. Strokes are the cause of vascular dementia.

A stroke, also known as a brain attack, occurs when a blood vessel in the brain ruptures or becomes clogged. This will cause the affected part of the brain not to get the blood it needs to function, and the affected area can die within minutes. Since dead brain cells are not replaced, the effects of the stroke may become permanent.

Transient Ischemic Attacks (TIAs), also known as mini strokes, are closely related to strokes. TIAs share many of the same symptoms as a stroke. The biggest difference between the two is the TIAs symptoms may last anywhere from five minutes to several hours. Because they do not last very long most people tend to ignore them. About one-third of all people who have a TIA will experience a stroke within two to five years after their first event.[33]

Look for the following symptoms:[34]

- Sudden weakness or numbness in the face, arm or leg, particularly on one side of the body
- Sudden confusion, difficulty understanding speech or trouble speaking
- Sudden trouble seeing out of one or both eyes
- Sudden trouble walking, including dizziness, loss of balance or lack of coordination
- Sudden severe headache with no known cause

When to Call 9-1-1

According to the Center for Disease Control (CDC), "Acting F.A.S.T. is Key for Stroke." Stroke treatments work best if the symptoms are recognized within the first three hours of symptoms occurring. If you think someone is having a stroke do the F.A.S.T. test:

- F—Face: Ask the person to smile. Does one part of their face droop?
- A—Arms: Ask the person to raise both arms. Does one arm drift downward?
- S—Speech: Ask the person to repeat a simple phrase, such as "See Spot run." Is their speech slurred or garbled?
- T—Time to call emergency services: If you see any of these signs, call 9-1-1 immediately.

Write down the time the symptoms first appeared because EMS will ask you. If you know the time the event first started, it will help them determine the best course of treatment for your loved one. Do not drive her to the hospital, let an ambulance transport her. EMS can start life-saving treatments right away—up to an hour sooner than if you take her by car. Time is of the essence when it comes to strokes.

Heart Attack

A heart attack happens when the blood supply to the heart is reduced or stopped.

When to Call 9-1-1

The American Heart Association lists the following possible warning signs of a heart attack:

- **Chest discomfort.** Most heart attacks involve discomfort in the center of the chest that lasts more than a few minutes – or it may go away and then return. It can feel like uncomfortable pressure, squeezing, fullness, or pain
- **Discomfort in other areas of the upper body.** Symptoms can include pain or discomfort in one or both arms, the back, neck, jaw, or stomach
- **Shortness of breath.** This can occur with or without chest discomfort
- **Other signs.** Other possible signs include breaking out in a cold sweat, nausea, or lightheadedness

Not all of these signs happen in every heart attack. Symptoms do vary widely between men and women. The most common sign with both men and women is chest pain, often for women it is between the shoulder blades. However, women are slightly more likely than men to have the other common symptoms, especially shortness of breath, nausea or vomiting, and back or jaw pain. If any of these symptoms occur or you even suspect a heart attack, call 9-1-1. Like strokes, time matters. People who arrive by ambulance usually get faster treatment at the hospital than those who arrive by car.

<u>Working with Emergency Medical Services</u>

Keep a duplicate medication list available in the event of an emergency. It should also include all drug allergies. The fire department or emergency medical technicians' (EMT) job will be much easier if they know what medications she is taking and when she takes them.

Print out a current copy of all the medications, stick it into a plastic sleeve and tape it into the inside of an overhead kitchen cabinet door, preferably one nearest the front door. Place a *red stick-on dot* on the outside of the cabinet door, so that any family member, caregiver, or EMT knows to look there first for this information. This is a common practice in assisted living facilities. If you are away from home, another family member may be there when your loved one needs emergency assistance, and this saves time when searching for information on blood thinners, pacemakers, or other crucial healthcare data.

The Personal Earthquake Bag Revisited

Your day will go a whole lot better if you are prepared for life's little emergencies. If you have already created your loved one's personal earthquake bag, it can come in very handy if you must go to the hospital. Once you have completed your loved one's care instructions for family and friends who are doing the respite care, the bag will save them from a lot of guess work.

When considering respite care, you might create a mini-personal earthquake bag, also known as a travel kit, designed for family members or friends who will be giving you respite, such as when taking your loved one out for a meal. (See *Emergency Preparedness*, page 40, or for an example travel kit see my website tracycramperkins.com/resources and select Useful Forms from the menu.)

How often you use the items in the personal earthquake bag will determine how often you need to replace them. Keep a check list of the items you keep in the bag. Check it once every month if you use it often or every three months if you don't use it regularly to make sure perishable items are fresh and you have enough supplies.

Planning ahead will save you time and energy that you can put into doing something fun. This way, you don't need to pack extra patience.

* * *

For additional resources and information, see *Appendices A*, page 210, and *B*, page 212.

Chapter 9: Travel, Vacations and Holidays

If all difficulties were known at the outset of a long journey, most of us would never start out at all. ~Dan Rather

This chapter covers the most common things to plan for when you are traveling or spending holidays with your loved one. There are two kinds of earthquakes in life: the kind that makes the ground shake below your feet and the kind that happens when your loved one does something unexpected because they are away from their normal environment.

When you travel with your loved one, you will need two types of Earthquake preparedness kits: one for a real disaster and one for day-to-day events that can happen with your loved one. Unexpected things will happen to your loved one away from home because they are out of routine. See *Emergency Preparedness*, page 40 for suggested items.

Why do you need a personal earthquake kit for travel? Think about your own health care. You have customized it with a regular routine for your environment, but those skills and supplies may not be useful or available in a new or different environment. It doesn't matter why your environment changes. It affects the way you take care of yourself.

For example, when a person without dementia transitions from work to retirement (positive), married to divorced (negative), childless to having a child (positive), how their day is structured will change. With dementia, it does not matter if the change is positive or negative, it will affect the way they behave in any given situation. They may not take good care of themselves, possibly gain or lose weight, or become the star of their own reality TV show with throngs of adoring fans. The results could be good, or they could derail your loved one.

Planning ahead may change a stressful experience into an enjoyable time for everyone involved.

Travel

Travel with your loved one is planned to be a positive experience, but it may not work the way you expect—and become a negative experience.

During the early stages of dementia, your loved one might still enjoy travel. There will come a time when travel may become too overwhelming. If you are planning a vacation which covers long distances, you need to evaluate the abilities, needs, and preferences of your loved one and their safety. Throughout this book I have stressed routine, routine, routine. Keep these things in mind when you are planning a trip:

- What is the best method of travel for your loved one? Car, train, bus, air, or motorhome?
    - If you chose air travel, can your loved one cope with airport security?
    - What about tightly scheduled connecting flights? Will you be able to stay with him or her at all times?
    - Does the airline offer a service to transport you and your loved one through the airport between gates for connecting flights?
    - Do they offer a quiet space if your loved one melts down between flights?
    - If your loved one melts down on the airplane, what will you use to distract her — music, a stuffed animal, a fidget quilt, snacks? What activity keeps her calm?
    - How will you handle toileting on the airplane?
    - If she is having issues with congested sinuses and plugged ears, can she tell you before you get on the plane to avoid ruptured eardrums?

Pick the mode of travel that provides the most comfort and least stress for the both of you.

- Choose a destination that is familiar to your loved one. Choosing a known destination will involve the fewest changes in daily routine. Pick places your loved one visited prior to the onset of dementia
- Changes in the environment may trigger wandering, even if the person is in the early stages of dementia. Coordinate with the rest of your party how you will keep your loved one safe. This might include a GPS tracker they wear as a watch or piece of jewelry
- Put together an itinerary that includes details about each place you plan to visit. Give copies to your emergency contact people at home. Keep a copy with you on the trip
- If you are staying in a hotel, let the staff know ahead of time your specific needs so they are prepared to assist you
- Bring your loved one's personal earthquake kit and double-check to make sure it is fully stocked. (See *Emergency Preparedness*, page 40.)
- Plan to travel during the time of day best suited to your loved one. Consider how holidays may impact your travel schedule and your loved one's state of mind. Traveling during the Thanksgiving holiday weekend or during Spring Break may not be the best choice. Do not rush. Creating a sense of urgency to get somewhere may cause your loved one to become agitated

- Plan your travel to match your loved one's routine as closely as possible. Match mealtimes, medication time, nap times. Whatever you can do to reduce wandering and behavioral issues will make your trip much more enjoyable

An example from my own life: We took my father on a cross country road trip which covered 4,000 miles by car. Every evening when sundowners set in, he could not understand how to use the hotel bathroom and confused the toilet for the sink. He would use the toilet water to brush his teeth if we weren't guiding him. After the first night, we purchased enough extra toothbrushes to cover each night we stayed in a hotel. It was earthquake preparedness on the fly.

In any room where the sink was located outside of the tub/shower and toilet area, he thought the bathroom was down the hall and attempted to leave the room when he needed to use the toilet. We needed extra devices to lock the hotel room door to prevent wandering. He knew how to remove the door chain, however, hotels with hinged bar locks confused him and prevented wandering.

Because of the rigors of travel, after you return from the trip, you may notice a decline in your loved one's cognition. If this happens, it will be permanent.

Vacations: Your Respite

Caregiver burnout is a reality for dementia caregivers, but it doesn't have to be. You need respite, down time, time to rejuvenate. If you plan on taking a vacation, whether it's a weekend getaway, a week or three, look into short-stay residential care for your loved one. In short stay settings your loved one receives medical care. They generally have activities available for your loved one's skill level.

When you schedule short stay care, there is a clear understanding of the duration your loved one will be under their care. Be aware that short stay care may stress your loved one. It is important there is enough skilled staff on hand to respond to your loved one's needs.

Some caregivers may not want to use this because they worry that if they give up care for even a short time, they will not be able to handle the burden of caregiving again. Respite care works better if you use it before you need it, before you hit the wall and burnout. Burnout can lead to elder abuse. You don't want to live with that burden.

There is generally no outside funding, such as insurance, that will cover short stay care. If you can't afford short stay care, check with family members who may be willing to care for your loved one while you are gone.

When you plan a vacation, make sure whoever is caring for your loved one and your emergency contacts have a detailed copy of your itinerary and a way to contact you.

Civic and Religious Holidays

Holidays and family reunions can be stressful, even for people without dementia. They become highly stressful for people with dementia. Look at it from their perspective. They are taken out of their normal routine, transferred to a new environment and asked to behave as though they are "normal." This will last for a short time, until their senses are saturated. They will be overwhelmed by the noise of multiple conversations, music, children playing, dishes clanking and possibly feeling crowded.

Then they will say something like, "I want to go home," or they will meltdown in front of everyone. This is a blessing in disguise. Because now everyone will be aware that something is wrong. They will recognize that perhaps their loved one is not doing as well as they imagine. It also opens the conversation about how to handle family gatherings differently.

According to Jolene Brackey, in her book, *Creating Moments of Joy Along the Alzheimer's Journey,* you may have to rethink holiday traditions. Have a family meeting to discuss what traditions must be included and what traditions are no longer needed. In the conversation include the following:

- Have a quiet room available when your loved one needs down time or a nap
- Consider spreading holidays out over several weeks or months. For example, if your family celebrates Christmas, then on Sunday, you go to the church service. Then over the next few weeks invite one family a week over for dinner. The next month open presents. If you spread it out over time, it will reduce the stress and increase the socialization your loved one receives
- If the caregiver is the one who traditionally prepares the family meals, you should change to a potluck with each family member or guest responsible for bringing something for the meal
- During the meal, make sure your loved one is sitting in their usual seat next to their favorite family member who can assist them
- Assign the person who is most attuned to your loved one's needs to make sure she is not left alone in a crowd. If she becomes restless, that person can take her for a walk or take her to her bedroom for a nap or some quiet time
- Make sure everyone knows your loved one needs something in her lap to distract her from the noise. It could be a beloved pet, a plush toy, a baby (or baby doll), a plate of finger food to nibble on or a blanket. Pair the item to your loved one's abilities

- Make sure everyone in the family knows to put your loved one and the caregiver first. *The rest of the family can adjust, the person with dementia cannot*
- Take turns spending time with your loved one during an event. This ensures other family members get quality time with your loved one and they can enjoy activities together, whether it is eating out, shopping, watching a ball game, or chatting. Make sure all family members are aware of your loved one's schedule and how to de-escalate disruptive behaviors (See *Distraction Techniques*, page 86)

It may take up to two weeks or longer for your loved one to recover from changes and the overstimulation of the outing. Which means you, the caregiver, will be dealing with the behavior issues that result until your loved one feels safe again.

Remember you represent safety, and their daily routine represents safety. Speeding up her recovery time could be doing something as simple as singing songs together, cuddling-up in a warm blanket with a cup of cocoa and watching an old movie, or laughter.

An example from my own life: When my father would act out after an outing with other family members. We figured out the trigger for his meltdown was the outing. The same behavior occurred each time he went out without us. We attempted coaching family members to be alert for his triggers. They did not always remember the triggers because it was not in their daily routine.

We paired down my father's behavior to three days for recovery from an outing with other family members because we stuck to his routine like nothing had happened to disrupt him. We emphasized the things that made him feel safe and loved. For him that routine meant repeating his favorite nursery rhymes, "kicking my butt" playing cards, and eating his favorite meals. During those three days he would lose his temper easily, yell obscenities, and if my husband wasn't home, he would throw things on the floor or against the wall. During those three nights, he would stand outside my bedroom door calling my name repeatedly until I got out of bed to help him. Thirty minutes later he would repeat the process and repeat and repeat—like a broken record—until morning.

On day four, we celebrated with a special treat. He didn't know why we celebrated, but he loved "the party." My treat that night—I spent quality facetime with my pillow and my pillow didn't care if I snored or drooled.

Chapter 10: Preparing Your Living Environment for Your Loved One

Looking Through Your Loved One's Eyes

In this chapter we will focus on preparing the living environment for your loved one. When we talk about something dementia-related, it will also relate to Alzheimer's Disease (A.D.). When we talk about something that is A.D. related it may not apply to dementia.

The way a memory impaired person relates to the world is different from the way you and I see, hear, smell, taste, or touch it. Their world will become increasingly unfamiliar. Imagine someone asks you to sit down in their family room, but you don't see the chair. You are hungry, and someone hands you a protein bar. But you don't know what it is. What about sitting in a restaurant with your family and becoming overwhelmed by the sounds—loud voices, clinking silverware, kitchen noise, a breaking glass, music, text message pings? What about smell? You smell your grandmother's apple pie baking in the kitchen, but where is the kitchen and where is Nana? You put change in your pants pocket and five minutes later you don't even know what it is you are feeling against your leg? What if you looked in the mirror and someone you don't know looked back at you?

You never know what someone is going through until you walk a mile in their shoes. Let's take a short walk together with Anita after she moved in with her son's family.

Anita's son, Jared, walked into her room Saturday morning. Tears rolled down Anita's soft, wrinkled cheeks. Her arms were wrapped around her waist. She rocked back and forth on the end of her bed. A sob escaped her lips.

Jared rushed to his mother's side taking her right hand in his, "Mom, what's the matter?" he asked.

What's Covered in This Chapter
- Looking Through Your Loved One's Eyes
- Safety First
  - Clutter
  - Lighting
  - Color Strategies Inside the Home
  - Flooring and Trip Hazards
  - Furniture and Interior Pathways
  - Bathroom Safety
  - Sound: What is that Noise?
  - Kitchen Safety
- Smell
- The Home Improvement Store is Your Friend
- Pharmacies, Medical Supply Stores or Used Medical Supply Stores
- Lock-up the following items in your home
- Telephone Tools

"There's someone watching me outside my window." Anita pointed toward the mirror above her dresser. She choked down another sob. *"She won't go away no matter what I do."*

"Mom don't be ridiculous, that's you in the mirror," Jared said. *"Come on, I'll show you."* Jared put his arm around his mother's shoulders.

She pushed him away. Shaking, her voice terse, she said, "Jared, I'm telling you there's a stranger outside my window. Why won't you believe me?"

Jared didn't understand his mother no longer recognized herself in the mirror. What Anita will remember is the anger, fear, and frustration her son caused. Who will have a rougher day with a combative family member? Jared. What could Jared do to calm his mother's fears the next time this happened? Her fear was real, it was her reality. The way to help her would be to enter her reality and walk her through to a place where she feels safe. He could walk in her shoes:

"There's someone watching me outside my window." Anita pointed toward the mirror above her dresser. She choked down another sob. *"She won't go away no matter what I do."*

Mom, I'll handle this." Jared put his arm around his mother's shoulder. *"Let's get you into a room where she can't see you and I will send her away."*

Jared walked his mother into the kitchen where his wife made breakfast. "Honey, someone is peeping into Mom's room. Can you stay with her while I take care of it?"

His wife nodded to Jared. She smiled at Anita. "Anita, would you like a glass of orange juice?"

Jared walked back into Anita's room and removed the mirror from the wall. He took the mirror to the garage. He wrapped it and put it in the attic.

When he walked back into the kitchen, Anita put down her glass of juice. Her voice quivered, "Is she gone?"

Jared smiled. "Mom, she won't ever come back. When you're ready, I'll walk you back to your bedroom. I want to make sure you're safe."

Anita smiled; her shoulders relaxed.

Does it matter that it was not real? Not in the least. What Anita will remember is not what Jared did, but the good feelings that he believed her, loved her, and supported her. Who is going to have a better day? Jared—and Anita.

Imagine how you would feel having all of your senses bombarded at once, while having greater difficulty separating yesterday from today. It might feel like riding on a speeding train while watching a tidal wave rush toward you. You have no control over what is going on around you.

When you plan a change in your living environment to adapt it for a memory-impaired person, the first question you want to ask yourself is, "Can I live with this change?" Another item to consider is if you make a change in his environment, will he be able to adjust to it? People with dementia can have trouble adjusting to even simple changes in their living environment.

With that said, some things to consider when preparing a home for someone with dementia are lighting, color strategies, flooring, furniture, and wall hangings, interior pathway obstructions and sounds. Keep in mind that no single suggestion will work in all situations.

If you want to hire contractors who specialize in aging-in-place construction the National Association of Home Builders has an online directory of certified specialists who can identify and/or do home modifications. Their website is: www.nahb.org/NAHB-Community/Directories. Choose "Professionals with Home Building Designations" and choose the filter for "CAPS."

Safety First

Whether you are caring for your loved one in their home or in yours, you need to make some changes to the environment to make it safer.

Alzheimer's Disease impairs a number of cognitive functions most of us take for granted. In increasing degrees, it reduces good judgement, behavior, and the ability to move through a familiar space.

Perhaps your loved one no longer remembers to turn off the stove, how to use the TV remote or the telephone. Eventually they may not remember their own belongings or where their bedroom is located, even if they have slept in the room for years. Once-familiar items become unfamiliar objects. Family members and life-long friends may cause them to be suspicious or afraid.

Striking the right balance can be a challenge. How do you know what is right? The mix will be different depending on the challenges the person with dementia exhibits.

Keep an eye on your loved one and see what he does within his environment. Does he talk to pictures on the wall or his reflection in the mirror? Does he become agitated like Anita when he does so? Does he grab items off the kitchen counter and examine them? Does he put his hands into the serving bowls instead of using a spoon or fork? Does he pick up the ketchup bottle or mustard and not know what to do with it? Does he have issues trying to figure out which utensil to use to eat his meal? Does he pick up everything on the bathroom counter, look at it, then put it down?

Using lighting, contrasting colors, moving or removing furniture, mirrors, wall hangings, and throw rugs can all help.

One size does not fit all, but the options below may help. They can be done over time based on budget constraints and the ever-changing needs of your loved one.

Clutter

Clutter or not to clutter—it shouldn't even be a question. As a person of clutter, I admit my mind works best in piles. However, the confusion caused by too much clutter in the home can create some unexpected and unpleasant surprises, including falls and choke hazards. But being too stark or barren reduces the visual stimulus needed for a person with dementia. The goal is to simplify and reduce the clutter to reduce confusion.

Lighting

The goal with lighting is to emulate daylight. With dimming eyesight, daylight lighting is the most soothing type of lighting for people with dementia.[35] As A.D. progresses, shadows may cause him to be afraid or not see items properly. Any glare combined with older eyes which do not adjust quickly to the lighting will add to the confusion. He may miss stair steps or walk into walls because he can't distinguish where the step ends and where the floor or wall begins. Because of glare or shadows or a monochromatic color scheme, he may not see a chair to sit in.

If you have fluorescent ceiling fixtures in your home, consider replacing any plastic or prismatic lenses with parabolic reflectors also known as parabolic grids. They look like a sheet of darkened, silver-coated, plastic squares. The reflectors diffuse the light and eliminate shadows.

If you use table or task lamps in his living space, use a single task lamp.[36] Having too many lamps in an area will create multiple shadows. Install lights in dark closets.

It may not be convenient to leave a hall light on in the evening, but neither is having to clean up after incontinence in the middle of the night because someone couldn't find the bathroom. If possible, consider using night lights to illuminate hallways from bedroom to bathroom—borrow an idea from the airlines: *"in the event of an emergency,"* or, in this case, preventing one. Use a roll of sticky-backed reflector tape to mark the path from his bed to the bathroom. Combine it with a cueing aid identifying the bathroom (See *Memory Aids and the Family*, page 29) so he can find it by himself.

Dimmer switches are another option that may help with the symptoms of Sundowners (a worsening of behaviors in the evening, see *Distraction Techniques*, Page 86), by raising the light levels as the sun goes down. Depending on the season and the person, "Sundowning" generally happens between 3 p.m. and 8 p.m.

Cordless window shades will help control the glare of early morning or late afternoon sun and may help with Sundowners. Using shades (roller or cellular) or blinds without cords in his bedroom will help him with his independence and reduce frustration and agitation caused by operating blinds with cords. When used in conjunction with hand-drawn drapes, you can block out most of the outdoor shadows.

Quick tip: Consider replacing floor lamps with wall mounted lighting. This will help reduce trip hazards. If you are in a rental property or apartment, consult your property manager or landlord before making any changes.

Color Strategies Inside the Home

Selecting a good color strategy in the home can help a person with A.D. navigate their environment by choosing contrasting colors. Studies have shown that color changes behaviors, positively and negatively for people with A.D.[37]

If you use different colors for different areas and spaces, it can help your loved one remain oriented to their living space and can help him get from room to room without getting lost within the home. For example, painting the bathroom door a different color, such as red or lime green, differentiate it from the rest of the doors in the living space making it easier to find, or exchange the door with a colorful shower curtain. Paint a half moon on the door. It's a symbol most of us recognize for an outhouse. Keep in mind using too much of one color, such as red can over-stimulate the mind, just as using too much of a cool color, such as blue, can under-stimulate the mind.[38]

Walk through each room of the home and look at the furnishings and the colors on the walls and floor. For instance, is the furniture in the family room in a light-colored wood? You may want to paint the walls a greenish-blue or warm apricot or peach. If the room has dark or varnished wood furniture, consider updating the walls with a light color to improve the contrast. [39]

If he has failing depth perception, bright contrasted colors can balance the gap in perception. Such uses could include using a contrasting color on the edges of kitchen cabinets to help your loved one orient themselves within the space and perhaps reduce accidents. Use flat paint rather than gloss to help eliminate glare and shadows. Avoid pastels unless you are disguising something you don't want your loved one getting into. Due to eyes yellowing and the thickening of the eye lenses with age, older people may perceive certain colors as washed out. When you add in dementia, the effect from using pastels makes them difficult to see.

Play with color on your computer before committing. Canva has a neat tool. Their Color Design Wiki gives information about different color combinations. It might help you with ideas. Their website: https://www.canva.com/colors/combinations/

Putting bright, colorful cushions on chairs may help him find his favorite chair within the living space. Consider putting bright colored frames on his favorite photos so he can find them on the walls. Get creative with brightly colored place mats or napkins under items he uses everyday like table lamps, the snack jars, cooking utensils, or the coffee pot.

Stairs can be an issue unless you use highly contrasting colors to mark the edge of each step. For example, a yellow stripe of tape on the lip of each step to reduce confusion of where one step ends, and another begins.[40]

The bathroom is an area which can create a lot of confusion. Consider painting the wall behind a white or light-colored toilet in a dark or contrasting color. If you can't change the wall color, replace the toilet seat with an alternate-colored seat. If you are using a mat at the base of your toilet, avoid the colors black or dark brown or dark blue. With these colors and failing perceptions, it will appear to be a hole in the floor or wall. Use a bright, contrasting color to liven up the floor and make it more obvious where the toilet is located.[41]

Black is your ally when you need to camouflage items to be avoided or prevent him wandering from home. Use black mats in front of every interior exit. Generally, when he sees what looks like a hole in front of the door, he will turn back from it without having to be guided. There is the possibility he may become scared for your safety if you walk across the door mat if he is focused on it.

In a similar vein, painting or wallpapering entry doors to match the surrounding walls makes them much harder to recognize. If you have glass doors, consider using window film artwork to disguise the glass. Pinterest is a great place to look for ideas if you search under "window film" or "wallpaper for windows." Full length draperies or curtains may also work to disguise doors.

Memory care facilities use wallpaper or painted scenes or designs on doors, including the elevator doors, to mislead residents with declining perception into thinking they are part of the wall, keeping the residents safe. If you enjoy wallpaper borders, consider placing a colorful border along the walls at waist height. Continue it across the door jamb and exit doors. You can also include contrasting, colorful arrows to point the way to the bathroom or the kitchen or his bedroom.

Quick Tip: Avoid using anything patterned with a checker pattern or polka dots or stripes of contrasting colors like black and white. They may be perceived as steps or holes in the floor. They may also be perceived as ants, spiders, or many other critters. If you want something that is not solid, choose items with simple geometric shapes or simple repeated designs like plaids or florals.[42]

Your loved one's sensitivity to color may change with the progression of their dementia, so it may be necessary to adjust the balance, brightness, or tones of colors as they progress through the disease.

Flooring and Trip Hazards

The Carpet Snake Advisory Board sent a reminder for their October conference. "Earn airline miles during the area rugs session: How to Have a Nice Trip. See you next fall."

Joking aside, fall risks increase as dementia progresses. When muscle loss progresses to a certain point, you will notice your loved one shuffling his feet. The number one cause of falls is floor coverings. Small pets can also be a trip hazard. Before you make any changes to your flooring, have his footwear checked.

The first time my father showed obvious issues walking, it turned out he did not have supportive shoes and his arches were falling. The shuffling was his way of compensating for the discomfort. If your loved one is diabetic, at the time of this writing, Medicare Part B will cover part of cost of the shoes—you pay 20 percent and the Part B deductible applies—if they are prescribed by a podiatrist, orthotist, prosthetist, pedorthist, or other qualified individual, such as a primary care physician (PCP).[43]

Keeping the flooring you have means keeping a few things in mind. Repair or level any uneven flooring. If you have carpet, remove area rugs. Make sure the carpet is secure. Keep in mind there will be more spills and accidents to clean up. If you have tile or linoleum flooring, keep it clean, but not shiny. Shiny floors create glare. They can create the illusion of ice or water in addition to possible slip hazards. Do not use tile or linoleum flooring that runs continuously up the wall. It will make it difficult for your loved to know where the floor ends and the wall starts.

Watch for shadows created by light coming in through windows. Adjusting the light level in the room using dimmer switches and/or adjusting any window coverings can compensate for shadows.

If you have a limited budget for new flooring, a laminate hardwood floor is ideal. It can be found at most large home improvement stores and is easy to keep clean. It tends to be the first choice of healthcare interior designers and architects who build facilities for the memory impaired.

For those who have the funds to do so, consider contacting a healthcare interior designer, accredited through the American Academy of Healthcare Interior Designers (AAHID), who specializes in dementia and A.D. environments. They may be able to add insights outside the scope of this book. Their website is: https://aahid.org/

Furniture and Interior Pathways

Keeping interior pathways clear of furniture, boxes, cords, and children's and pet's toys will help your loved one successfully and safely navigate through the home. He will gain a sense of accomplishment being able to find the bathroom, kitchen, and perhaps his favorite chair with fewer issues.

As his motor skills diminish, balance will become more of an issue. Furniture should be simple and sturdy. Remove any furniture that is difficult to get out of. For example, chairs should have sturdy arms, so he can push himself upright. Most women require shorter chair seat depth. Overstuffed furniture can also cause difficulties getting up. Remove rocking chairs because they can tip over. However, a glider, also known as a platform rocker, is a safe option. It will mimic the motion of a rocking chair without the risk of falling over.

Keep in mind furniture that wobbles will appear to a memory impaired person like the furniture is about to fall over. Using sticky-back felt pads can help stabilize a piece of furniture. Built-in shelves are a safer alternative to free-standing shelves. They are a great way to keep the area clutter free (See *Memory Aids and the Family*, page 29) and help your loved one find cherished items. If you do use free-standing shelves, be sure to anchor them to a wall stud with furniture earthquake anchors or straps.

Keep wall hangings simple. Mirrors—wall mounted, handheld or as table decoration, should be removed from areas your loved one inhabits when he is near the middle stage of Alzheimer's Disease. If he is having a nice conversation with his reflection, no one is being harmed, leave the mirrors. When he shows symptoms of agitation remove the mirrors. The mirrors will create the illusion someone is watching him, perhaps a long-lost parent or an intruder as was the case with Anita at the beginning of this chapter.

Keep fish tanks out of reach. While watching the fish may be very soothing, the combination of glass, electrical pumps and potentially poisonous aquatic life could be dangerous to a curious person with A.D.

Bathroom Safety

When inspecting the bathroom, make sure it is free of safety hazards that could potentially cause injury.

Here are a few things to consider:

1. Is the door a pocket door? If it does not have a doorknob, they will not be able to figure out how to open it.
2. Is the floor clear of clutter that could cause a fall? Even a scale can be a trip hazard.

3. Is the floor level and non-slippery? Is there a wax coating on the floor? If so, remove it.

4. Are there safety rated grab bars next to the toilet or in the tub/shower area? If not install them. Towel bars will not prevent a person from falling.

5. Can he safely get up or sit down on the toilet? If not consider a raised toilet seat. Commode liners are available to ensure urine and feces goes into the toilet. Do his feet touch the floor when he sits on the raised seat? If not, consider adding a toilet stool similar to a Squatty Potty for stability.

6. Is the tub/shower floor nonslip? If not, install nonslip mats or stickers or decals

7. Is the bathtub spout cushioned? If not, purchase a foam cover to help reduce injury from a fall. They are available in most medical supply stores and in retail baby departments.

8. Is the tub/shower large enough to hold a bath chair? A chair will help you bathe him safely. Measure your tub's interior and exterior width, and then go online to check bathing chair dimensions. There are bathing chairs available with drop arms, so if you are transferring someone in a wheelchair it will ease the transfer. Most shower chairs are white. If your walls are white or light colored, consider putting a colored towel on the seat the help him find it.

9. Is he too heavy or too big for you to lift him into and out of the tub? There are devices such as a bath lift or a slider chair. They are not cheap and can cost as much as $3,000. However, they are less expensive than remodeling your home. In the long run they will pay for themselves because you will not have to pay a professional caregiver to come in and do the bathing for you.

10. Is the water temperature too hot? If so, change the setting on the water heater to 120 degrees Fahrenheit (49°C) or lower to prevent scalding. Please note that A.D. patients may not perceive temperature in the same way you do. What feels comfortable to you may be too hot for him. Have him check the comfort level of the water before getting into the bath. This too will diminish over time and he won't be able to tell you if something is too hot or too cold. Watch him for changes in skin color such as skin flushing for too hot, or blue lips or shivering for too cold.

11. What kind of flush toilet do you have? He may not be able to use a two-flush system toilet. You may need to install a toilet tank with handle. If he has arthritis, this is a must.

12. What kind of faucet does your bathroom sink have? Consider getting a lever-style faucet or tap turners, especially if your loved one has arthritis.

13. Are the faucets clearly labeled for hot and cold? Are the labels correct?

For guidelines to properly installing items like grab bars and other bathroom safety features, visit ADABathroom.com. http://www.adabathroom.com/index.html

Sound: What is that Noise?

Sound is also a part of our everyday lives. While we take it for granted and can sort out or ignore the sounds around us, your loved one may become overwhelmed when barraged with too much sound all at once. As the disease progresses, they may not only experience hearing loss, but also the ability to recognize, or recognize and "tune-out" the background noise they hear.

Additionally, there is a strong correlation between hearing loss and progressing dementia.[44] Many of the symptoms of hearing loss are similar to those of Alzheimer's disease (see *Doctors, Pharmacists and Me, Oh My*, page 53). Which means the sounds of the television, cell phones, loud music, flushing toilets, running water, traffic, playing children, or multiple conversations can agitate him. Watch him for signs that he can't understand what is being said to him or is becoming agitated by the conversations going on around him. For example, is he making grunting noises or repeatedly standing up and sitting down? If you touch him on the arm, get eye contact, and speak to him, is there a change in behavior?

Can you move him to a quiet space within your home? Can you play music he enjoys? Make sure the sound is at a level appropriate for your loved one to hear it, but not so loud you want to rip your ears off. If you want to speak to him turn off the music or television to limit distractions. Make sure the rest of the family knows to do this.

Are you talking over the top of him or around him during a meal? Is there a place where he can eat in peace and silence without other noises or movements disturbing him and distracting him from eating?

Some things to consider with noise reduction especially at night, watch his behavior for clues to what works for him.[45]

- Do you have things on the wall that absorb sound, reducing echo? Sound absorbing curtains or fabric wrapped acoustical panels or artwork on the wall may absorb sound. If you are more Avant Garde in your decorating perhaps incorporating sound proofing foam will reduce echoes too
- Be careful with floor coverings such as area rugs, they pose a trip hazard even if secured by tape. Consider installing a floating floor out of laminate or engineered hardwoods to absorb sound
- Do your lights buzz, either fluorescent or LED? Consider replacing the ballast or starter on a fluorescent fixture or replacing a LED fixture that buzzes. A qualified electrician can install them if you don't have the time or experience

- Do you run your dishwasher or washer and dryer at night? How does he react to those noises over time?
- Do you have children running in and out of the house slamming doors?
- Check for air passages around doors and windows and seal them. You may not notice the noise, but he might
- If you have exposed walls made up of concrete, brickwork or plasterboard, they can create echoes and confusion. Consider covering them with something which will absorb sound
- Do you have loud ticking clocks? Do the water pipes rattle when the toilet is flushed? Do you have a central heating system with a whole house fan that turns on and off?
- Is he disturbed by the sounds of meal preparations?
- If he wears hearing aids, are they clean and working? There is a possibility of delirium when he can't hear[†]

Do not underestimate the power of silence when he is agitated. It may help him focus and regain control of his emotions.

[†]Delirium appears as a worsening of dementia symptoms. For example, they can't focus and have difficulty maintaining or shifting their attention. They may speak incoherently and have issues either staying awake or they become restless and agitated. Delirium usually goes away when the symptoms are treated.

For more ideas see *Distraction Techniques, Meltdown Trigger List*, page 102.

Kitchen Safety

The kitchen contains many areas where accidents can happen. A person with dementia may not remember to turn off the stove, may put an empty pan on a hot burner, or may hide items under the burners. Depending on the type of stove you have, you can remove the knobs for the burners or install timers on the stove or microwave or you can have an electrician add a switch hidden in a cupboard or other area not visible to the person with dementia which will cut the power to the stove and electrical outlets. If you choose to turn the stove's power on and off at the circuit breaker—it is not designed like a light switch. Keep in mind it will shorten the life of the circuit breaker and the handle may break off in your hand.

He may no longer remember how to use a knife and cause himself serious injury. Consider placing all sharp objects in a drawer and add a childproof lock to the drawer. Remove all clutter on the counter. If he believes he is still hungry after a meal because he doesn't remember eating, he may mistake small objects on the counter for food and eat them. Instead, leave out finger foods he can nibble on such as carrots, celery, crackers, cheese cubes, or olives.

For more suggestion on what to remove, see *Lock Up the Following Items in Your Home* on page 84.

Smell

Our sense of smell is very powerful. We can recognize over one trillion odors.[46, 47] It is the only sense which has a direct route to the brain. All of our other senses are routed through our thalamus (a part of the brain above the brain stem).

Smells can affect him in a deep way, whether good or bad. Many Alzheimer's care facilities use aroma therapy to evoke fond memories. The following essential oils are thought to help people with dementia:[48]

- Basil
- Chamomile
- Coriander
- Lavender
- Lemon
- Neroli (distilled from the flowers of the Seville orange)

Researchers have found reduced levels of agitation and distress in dementia patients with the use of essential oils.[49] Aromatherapy can be used in a number of ways:

- Baths—adding a few drops to the water
- Inhalation and vaporizers
- Massage—applying directly to the skin

Consider contacting an aromatherapist to assist in choosing the correct therapy for your loved one.

The Home Improvement Store is Your Friend

There are many devices that can be used in the home for safety and are available through most home improvement stores and their websites. For example:

- Emergency Power-Failure LED Lights
- Hand-held shower head
- Door alarms
- Double sided tape or other skid-proofing for area rugs
- Timer for outdoor lights
- LED lighting
- Safety Rated Grab Bars
- Smoke and carbon monoxide detectors

- Childproof plugs for unused electrical outlets
- Automatic shut-off switch on stove
- Hide-a-key rock or lockbox, in case your loved one locks you out of the house
- Non-skid strips for the floor

If you have staircases in your home, baby gates may help keep him from climbing stairs by himself, especially if there is a risk of falling.

Closets you do not want him scavenging in can also present a problem. If closet doors have knobs, you can install childproof locks. These locks do not have keys, but they require dexterity to open, which will be too complicated for someone with dementia. Install the locks or childproof drawer latches where you keep hazardous household cleaners, medicine cabinets, the junk drawer, or other drawers anywhere you don't want him to explore. People with A.D. are at higher risk of eating small objects like matches, hardware, plastic, erasers, etc. The junk drawer is an opportunity waiting to be tasted.

Preventing your loved one from walking out of the house might take more than changing the color of the door or covering it. There are several other options which might help, such as changing the door handle from active to passive (meaning it won't turn) or using loose fitting doorknob covers and putting a dead-bolt or active handle either at the top or bottom of the door. If you have small children, the top of the door is preferred. Adding a door alarm to alert you when a door is opening or closing, can also add peace of mind. It can be as simple as the doorknob decorations with jingle bells sold around the winter holidays or a battery powered door alarm or the alarm system in your home.

Pharmacies, Medical Supply Stores, or Used Medical Supply Stores

There are items which may not be available through a home improvement store or their website, but will make your life easier as a caregiver:

- Shower Chair
- Cane
- Walker
- Wheelchair
- Blood Pressure Cuff
- Mediscope (used for checking eyes, ears, and throat for signs of infection)
- First Aid Supplies
- Pill minders
- Incontinence Supplies
- Nonslip bathtub mats or stickers

- Dycem nonslip material (It can be used to stabilize material like glasses filled with liquids, used to open jar lids or to keep objects from rolling. It is reusable, easy to peel from any surface and can be cleaned with soap and water.) It comes in multiple colors, including red and blue that can double as a cueing aid to orient your loved one to an item. Do not use black with any item your loved one uses
- Grab bars
- Raised toilet seat or raised safety toilet seat with handles
- Lap Buddy (a piece of foam that sits across the lap and is tucked under the arms of the chair. Used with people who can no longer walk safely un-attended and shouldn't wander. It's easier for you to remove than a belt restraint.)
- Egg-crate foam (used for adjusting the position of a person who is wheelchair or bed bound to prevent pressure or bed sores) or bedsore rescue cushions

Check with Medicare, Medicaid, or supplemental insurers to see if they will cover the expense for any of these supplies.

With the progression of dementia will come a time when you will need to lock up items that could pose a danger to someone with decreased judgement.

Lock Up the Following Items in Your Home

- Alcohol
- Bathroom items like toothpaste, shampoos, soap, perfume, lotions, rubbing alcohol, or hydrogen peroxide†
- Cleaning and household products like paint thinner, matches, lighters, or laundry detergent pods†
- Foods like spices, sugar, and salt if you see him putting too much on food
- Gasoline cans and other dangerous items in the garage
- Guns and other weapons such as scissors, knives, power tools, and machinery
- Hide plastic bags, they may be a choke hazard to someone with A.D.
- Prescriptions and over-the-counter medicines
- Remove poisonous plants†

†Contact the National Poison Control Center at 1-800-222-1222 or www.poison.org for information on which plants are poisonous, household chemicals, detergent pods, or any other potentially dangerous substance.

For further information on this topic, visit the National Institute on Aging at https://www.nia.nih.gov/health/home-safety-and-alzheimers-disease

Telephone Tools

There will come a time when your loved one will not remember telephone calls they received or what they were about. Tools to help with this are Caller ID so you can scan through the incoming call list. This will not help with masked phone numbers from scammers. For landlines, you can set up an answering machine to record all telephone calls. This may also be helpful in the event of scammers calling.

Register his phone number on the National Do Not Call Registry to reduce the number of solicitations calls he receives. Their website: www.donotcall.gov.

His memory of telephone numbers will disappear with the advancement of dementia. Keep a list of emergency contacts near the phone, include 9-1-1 and the Poison Control Center 1-800-222-1222. Make sure it is in print large enough he can read it without glasses.

There will come a time when he might not recognize you and call 9-1-1 every night because there is a stranger in his home or in his bed. A simple solution is to disguise the telephone. For example, use a decorated box or a decorative hollowed-out book to hide the phone. If you use a cell phone exclusively, change the password to something he will not remember, or use a phone which unlocks using your fingerprint, a pattern, or facial recognition.

For those of you caring for a significant other where you still share a bed, if disguising the telephone does not work, try this when he does not recognize your face: once he's in bed turn out the light. Leave your bedroom for a few minutes, then come to the door and announce you are whoever he is expecting to join him in bed. He may not recognize you with the light on, but he will recognize your voice well into the disease.

* * *

For longer lists of supplies, refer to *Appendix B*, page 212.

Chapter 11:
Distraction Techniques

"This life is a test — it is only a test. If it had been an actual life, you would have received further instructions on where to go and what to do." ~Anonymous

In this chapter we will focus on your loved one's reactions or over-reactions to situations. When we talk about something dementia related it will also relate to Alzheimer's Disease (A.D.). When we talk about something that is A.D.-related it may not apply to dementia. There are several things you can do for your loved one and for yourself as they walk the path of decline.

We will look at possible solutions for certain behaviors that can and will cause issues. It may sound easy when you read it,

but when you are faced with an angry or frightened loved one you may panic if you are not prepared. Advanced knowledge of the possibilities ahead of you is empowering.

An example from my own life: My father's favorite form of exercise every morning was trimming back the overgrown Salal hedge in our front yard while chatting with the neighborhood walkers. He wielded my grandfather's garden shears with an artist's touch. He would pick up the fallen branches with a flourish and drop them in the blue yard waste bin for his audience. The neighbors would then ask him to work on their yard. He posed with the yard waste bin and soaked up the praise.

One Saturday after breakfast while I washed the dishes, my father volunteered to take out the trash for me. After lunch, my husband, father, and I went grocery shopping. When we returned home, some fir branches lay across our driveway. Each one of us grabbed some branches. I opened the yard waste bin. There sat the trash bag, its red ties waving at me from the top of the yard waste bin. I laughed.

I pulled the garbage bag out of the yard waste bin.

My father yelled, "Stop what you're doing," his voice low and threatening.

My spine tingled, and my stomach hit bottom. I reverted to my 10-year-old self in trouble for wasting food by using an entire box of Grape Nuts for pixie dust.

I faced my father. He charged at me, wielding a branch in his hand. My husband threw himself between us. Crashing into my much larger husband was enough to stop him. His face bright red, he threw the branch on the ground and yelled, "I want to fix it."

I stepped out of the way. He grabbed the bag from my hand and put it in the waste bin while cursing himself for his own stupidity. In that moment, I realized the depth of his loss.

I did not consider his feelings when I laughed about the bag. With my back to him, I did not see his body language change when I escalated the situation from calm and happy to aggressive. His Alzheimer's Disease had progressed to a place where he used the yard waste bin as his catch all. In consideration of his feelings, I moved the mistargeted trash and recycling to the correct bins when he was not present, so he wouldn't feel slapped-in-the-face.

Practicing the following distraction techniques ahead of time will make it easier to cope when an unexpected situation charges at you.

I Want to Go Home

Sometime during the moderate stage of dementia, you may hear the phrase, "I want to go home," even if your loved one has lived in the same house for 30 years. Or if she has been relocated to a new living environment, she may not recognize it as "her home," or she may be telling you she is not comfortable in her environment. Time works differently in a confused brain, so she may have lived someplace many years and only think she has been there a few hours or even a day. You should also know that if you relocated someone with moderate dementia, it could take up to six months or more for them to adjust to their new living environment.

Look at the "I want to go home" scenario from her point of view, depending where she is in her dementia, she may think she is in her twenties, not her seventies. When she looks around the room, she doesn't see her "home," she sees a strange place she's never been before. She might be worried about her kids coming home from school, her husband wondering where she is, making dinner for her family, who's taking care of her animals, or her mom waiting for her to come home.

In her confusion, telling her, "No, you live here now," or "This is your home," will cause her to think you are lying. She will panic and try to escape. She only knows what she sees in front of her. You are not in her reality. You will need to join her where she is.

This is where redirecting her comes in very handy. Instead of correcting her, let her choose to stay.[50] For example:

- How about some lunch (or dinner) first?

- I made dessert for you; would you like some dessert?
- Let's get you dressed before you go.
- I need your help with [insert activity here].
- [Insert name she would understand, her church, PTA members, any organization she volunteered for that might make a free meal] **made us** [insert favorite meal]. It would be impolite for her to leave a free meal.
- What is your favorite thing about home? or Tell me about your home? For example, she might not be feeling comfortable in her surroundings, and this may give you a clue what needs to be addressed.

If it is happening around 3:30 p.m. every day, and she's telling you the kids will be coming home from school, figure out where you, if you are her child, or her kids were when school would get out and let her know that:

- [Insert your name here] is staying at [name of best friend—someone she trusts] house for dinner.
- [Insert your name or a sibling's name here] has: band practice, soccer, football, job at fast food restaurant. Whatever you or your siblings would have been doing after school including sleep overs. For all she knows every night is Friday night.
- If she is looking for her spouse, be very specific and say things like:
    - [Insert spouse's first name here] is working late tonight on the [insert project name]
    - [Insert spouse's first name here] called, he is having a beer [or insert other activity he did] with [insert one of his friend's name's here]
    - [Insert spouse's name here] is at bowling league this evening. Or whatever hobby she would remember that she would not attend with him

If she is worried about her parents or husband or kid(s) wondering where she is, let her know her [mom or dad, spouse, you] just called and said it was too dark for her to walk home this evening. What this does is gives her permission to relax because "they" know where she is in this moment.

When working with men, they have different motivations. They are much more difficult to get to stay. If redirecting them with food doesn't work, they want to work and be useful, so you need to be a bit more creative.

- Ask him for help moving something "heavy"
- Ladies: take his arm after "you" have made the above request and walk with him. He may be so distracted to be walking a woman down the hall, he will even forget about moving the box
- Ask him his opinion on fixing something that is broken. Perhaps he worked on cars, or was a plumber, or whatever profession or hobby he preferred

It is very common for both men and women to pack to go home. It can be very disturbing for you and make you feel guilty enough to move your family member back home to take care of them. Then once they are home, they may be so disoriented they still want to go home. Yet the reason which caused you to place your loved one in the care facility still remains.

An example from my own life: My mother had dementia and was in the last stages of cancer. The morning after we moved my mother into a hospice care facility, I came over to check on her. She was out of bed, fully dressed, wearing make-up, styled her hair, and packed her bags. She told me she was ready to go home. I had not seen her out of bed except in a wheelchair in nearly a year.

I stared at her for a moment while my mind derailed like a bullet train flying off a damaged bridge at 200 m.p.h. *How did she do that?*

I made the mistake of blurting out, "You are home."

She grabbed the back of the chair next to her and bent over like I'd gut punched her. Tears spilled from her eyes; her face turned pale. She repeated over and over, "That can't be right. Did your father leave me?"

At the time, I did not have the knowledge to redirect her to spare her feelings.

None of us is perfect. We all make mistakes, and we can learn from them. If you make a mistake, forgive yourself so you can move forward and put what you learn to good use. Then let your family, friends, and any other caregivers know what works so they can use it too.

Shadowing

Shadowing is when your loved one follows you around the house imitating what you are doing or becomes angry when you want some time to yourself. Why does this occur? You represent safety. She will come to rely on you to keep her from getting embarrassed or becoming frustrated and to help her fill in the blanks for those things she can't remember. This may present itself with her constantly interrupting what you are doing or her repeating the same phrase or activity over and over.

This behavior generally occurs in the late afternoon or early evening. It can drive you into your pillow to muffle a scream.

If you want to modify the behavior, pay attention to the following environmental factors:

- What behavior does she exhibit prior to her shadowing you?
- Does it happen around the same time every day?
- What is happening in the house when the behavior begins?
- Are you making dinner?

- Helping the kids with their homework?
- Cleaning?
- Preparing for company?
- Have you noticed anything that breaks the cycle? Like giving her tasks of her own, such as stacking magazines, dusting, folding laundry, or setting the table for dinner? It may help redirect her
- If your house is noisy in the later afternoon or early evening, music, audiobooks, or television may be a good distraction in an area where there won't be other noises
- If your living space is limited, ask her if she will accept the use of headphones to block out the household background noise to aid her in listening to something she prefers. The bonus: you don't have to listen to the same thing 45 times in one week
- Try distracting her with an Alzheimer's "busy apron," "twiddle muff," "fidget quilt," or "fidget sleeves." They are available online, or you can make your own. Check Pinterest for ideas
- Try using a baby monitor to talk to her from another room
- Did using positive phrases work well for her? For example, "I love you," or "Thank you for setting the table [or insert other activity here], I really appreciate it," or "That [insert outfit name] looks great on you."

<u>Note these in the meltdown trigger list and share them with your family and friends.</u>

Use the Meltdown Trigger List, explained below, to track the behaviors for a few days to identify the common incident(s) which provokes the behavior.

If she panics when you are out of the room, even for a short time, consider using a baby monitor. You can talk into the monitor while you are doing chores around the house and she can hear your voice or even respond. If you are trying to shower, try putting a timer next to her and telling her that once she hears the alarm go off, you will be back. Use a cueing aid next to the timer reminding her where you went and when you'll be back. When you come back announce that you kept your word and were back when the timer rang.

Try not to show annoyance. Your life will be smoother if you are the calming, smiling influence, no matter how you feel. Develop a handful of positive phrases like "You look marvelous today," or "I love you," or "It's a beautiful day today," or whatever feels natural for you. Your repeating certain uplifting phrases often works well for most dementia sufferers.

Make sure there are enough daily activities to channel her energies. It might be working in the yard, like my father, or folding laundry. If she volunteered, perhaps stuffing envelopes. Think back to the time before she had dementia, what did she used to do when you were growing up? It doesn't matter if she does the same thing every day or repeats an activity two, three, or more times a day. The object is to make her feel useful. Whatever she does, don't "fix it" for her if it's not done properly. Who cares if the cups are where the plates should be or if the forks are scattered around the table? This is not about teaching a child how to set the table; it's about empowering an adult who is now lost at sea with no hope of ever seeing the shore again. Compliment her on a job well done and your nerves will be a little less frayed by the end of the day.

Make sure you arrange some sort of respite time for yourself every few days. Having an adult follow you everywhere, sometimes mimicking what you are doing, sometimes repeating everything you say without a break is exhausting. Even if your caregiving break is only for an hour or two, a break can be energizing. Give yourself some personal time. Invite a family member or close friend to come over and stay with her while you have a cup of coffee and share a tee hee moment with another friend, get some shopping done, or sit in a park and soak up the sun. We all need a little bit of privacy. She will adapt well enough to someone else visiting her for a short time, and socializing is good for her, too.

Sleep Schedule Changes from Night to Day

Dementia sufferers, especially those with A.D., will have sleep disruption as the disease progresses. According to the Alzheimer's Association, those with late-stage A.D. spend up to 40 percent of their time lying awake in bed at night. My own father had issues with his sleep schedule changing from sleeping at night to sleeping during the day.

To combat this issues, there are a few things you can try and a few things to avoid.

Avoid using sleeping pills with someone who has dementia. It increases their fall risk and can leave them with a "hung-over" feeling, worsening their behaviors, including irritability. It is better to try non-drug related options for improving sleep before choosing to use a prescription medication.[51] Avoid both caffeine and alcohol.

Keep your loved one engaged in activities like adult day care, exercise, outings with family or friends, take them on simple errands. Anything that will keep her walking and moving. When she shows signs of fatigue, a quick nap is in order. Limit napping during the day to twenty or thirty minutes at a time as needed. It is tempting to let her sleep for three hours so you can have some down time, but you will pay for it when you want to sleep at night. Stick to her daily routine.

Unfortunately, she will not sleep all night. If she wakes up in the middle of the night, don't force her back into bed, find a simple activity for her so she can relax and become tired. It could be watching television, sorting buttons, or listening to an audio book or old radio program.

Inability to Make Decisions

At some point, most likely occurring in the moderate stage, she will be unable to make a decision. Decision making requires the ability to remember likes and dislikes and deciding how she feels about it right then. The ability to juggle several preferences in a few moments to make the decision is easy with a healthy brain. If she can't remember what food she likes or what clothing to wear for the weather outside, she may become overwhelmed, anxious, and frustrated.

For a person with Alzheimer's Disease, each decision, no matter how small, like where can I sit, can cause her to be afraid of making what might be the wrong choice, or she just can't remember where to sit or recognize places to sit.

When decision making difficulties occur try one of these _after_ a choice has been offered:[52]

- Give her time to make a decision. Remember if she feels rushed, she might become anxious

- If she is having trouble making a decision after a minute or two, share a suggestion with her. For example, after asking would you like to wear the red dress or the blue dress, say something like, "The blue dress sure brings out the color in your eyes." Or if you are at a restaurant try "I'm having [insert food name], do you want that too?"

- Reduce the number of overall choices. If you go to a restaurant, do not go to a buffet, it will be overwhelming, and she might take food out of the serving trays with her bare hands. Keep fewer clothes in her closets and drawers. Have duplicates of all her favorite clothing because once an item is lost, she may accuse you of stealing it. Even though you didn't lose it, you can apologize for losing it and be the hero when you "return" it

- Limit choice to no more than three items. If you know she loves strawberry ice cream, and that is one of the flavors, suggest it last. Many times, she will accept the last thing she hears. If she appears confused, suggest her favorite. Keep in mind her sense of taste and smell will change over time and so might her favorite foods

- With clothing, once you've learned her preferences, you can always place the preferred clothing on the top where she will "choose" it first

- For an activity to help with Sundowners (a worsening of behaviors in the evening), put a spare set of her favorite clothes in a box without her seeing the content of the box. Next ask her to help wrap it as a gift for a friend. The next morning leave it on her bed. Everyone enjoys receiving presents. She will start out the day feeling good and wear her new clothing. You will now have an opportunity to wash her dirty clothing. Heh-heh-heh
- Don't take away all her choices. She will feel empowered when she can choose between two items. However, when she shows you it is too overwhelming, take a step back and do not rush her

Hallucinations

There are a host of items to think about when someone is having a hallucination. Did she start any new medication? Have you had her pharmacist do a drug interaction check? (See *Doctors, Pharmacists and Me, Oh My*, page 60.) Are the curtains in her bedroom closed at night? If yes, are there shadows from moving branches or a neighbor's flapping flag? Patterns on the chairs, floors, or walls can create the illusion of spiders, insects, snakes or many other critters.

Hallucinations are generally visual, but they can also come in the form of other senses, such as smell or sound.

With television and mirrors, there is the possibility of hallucinations. She may think the people on the screen are real or her reflection is someone else. Hallucinations require patience. No matter what the cause, treat it like it is real.

Logical explanations will not work because two or more parts of her brain are dying.

Take a deep breath and follow the hallucination through to its logical conclusion. The more you immerse yourself in her reality, the better the outcome.

An example from my own experience, one evening after a long day out with us, my father retired to his room to watch TV before dinner. He fell asleep watching the Encore Western Channel with the remote in his hand. In his sleep, he accidentally changed the station to the History Channel showing a WWII battle reenactment. He woke up seeing the carnage.

He rushed into the kitchen. Sweat rolled down the side of his blanched face. He said, "We've gone to war, it's on our street. We need to get somewhere safe."

I asked, "Did you see it on the news?"

"Outside my window."

"Can I peek?"

He nodded.

He followed me to his bedroom. His voice cracking, "Tracy, stay below the window."

The window shade was down. Fortunately, there was a commercial on the TV that did not belong on Encore Westerns when we walked in. I casually picked up the remote from his bed when I knelt below window level. I hit the previous channel button and dropped the remote. I kept below the windowsill and lifted the shade about two inches. My father crawled up next to me. We both peeked outside. Our neighbor blew leaves off her driveway.

He said, "She doesn't know she's in danger. We have to go out there and warn her."

We went outside. My neighbor's mother had A.D., so my neighbor had first-hand experience coping with hallucinations. She assured him she was fine. He relaxed, but he spent three days peeking out the window before he resumed normal behavior.

Once you have walked your loved one through to the conclusion of the hallucinations, reassure her she is safe.

Keep in mind that even if you carry a hallucination out to its logical conclusion, the fear that triggered it may not go away. You may have repeated episodes with the same type of hallucination.

Sometimes you may need some creative help. If she is seeing insects crawling on the walls when you don't, ask if you can help. If she agrees, then have a friend or neighbor put on a "uniform" and exterminate what she is seeing. Ask her to point out anything that may have been missed.

If she is seeing a person in the room that you don't, do not leave her by herself in the room. It will only escalate the situation. Be honest, tell her you can't see them, but you know she can. Acknowledge she is upset. Ask if you can sit down with her. Reassure her you will stay until the person is gone. Remember, this is very real to her.

Take deep breaths in and let them out slowly between each reassuring sentence telling her that she is safe, and you won't leave her. She will begin to mimic your breathing. Once she is calmer, consider creating funny scenarios together in which you get rid of the intruder, like bouncing the stranger out of the room on a hippety-hop, paper mâché them to the garbage truck, or spraying the stranger with Silly String. Make it lighthearted and ridiculous, so you can both have a laugh together. The safer and happier she feels, the better your day will be.

If you are taking care of a man, keep in mind, he will be more responsive to someone in uniform. Do you have a male friend or neighbor who can wear a uniform that meets the hallucination, such as a cable repair man, security guard, policeman, or fireman? Or a male friend who radiates calm and confidence, and can come in to fix his day? Men are more receptive to fellow males fixing the problem or issue.

Hallucinations can also be a symptom of delirium. Delirium hallucinations are a sign of an infection or pain. Be sure to mention the hallucinations to her primary care physician to rule out medical causes.

When you are having a difficult day, so is she. If you just tell her, "There is no one in your room," or say, "I'll take care of it," then do nothing, she might call 9-1-1.

If you don't want to deal with her hallucination, ask yourself, "If this were happening to me, how would I feel if no one believed me and everyone refused to help?"

This is the time to use a distraction technique where you call a friend to come over to act as the exterminator. Help is there if you ask for it. Don't be afraid to ask. Besides, watching your friend—dressed in a uniform—killing imaginary bugs may just put a smile on your face.

Delusions

Delusions, also known as paranoid delusions, occur in someone with dementia because they have lost the ability to make good judgements. With a mind which cannot reason, she might blame others for any difficulty she is having. If she loses her glasses, she may accuse you of stealing them. If she doesn't recognize the neighbor mowing her lawn, she might think it is someone sneaking around with her husband.

The most common delusions are spousal adultery, stealing, belief that an intruder is invading their home, or claiming an imposter replaced a family member. They can happen in any stage of A.D. but are most common during the moderate stage—a time when the brain's ability to recognize reality deteriorates.

Here are the don'ts and do's with delusions:

- Don't try to prove your innocence when accused of stealing. The more you protest, the more the delusion becomes fixed in her mind
- Do let her vent her frustrations. Listen to her and give emotional support. Don't you feel better when someone listens to you?
- Don't try to berate her for accusing you. Again, it will confirm her suspicions
- Do encourage her to give you details by asking questions. For example, if it's an intruder, ask where the intruder went. If there is money involved, ask her when she first noticed it was missing. Regarding money, if she's used to having credit cards or money in her wallet, put a few dollars in her wallet or an inactive credit card or gift card
- Don't agree with the delusion, it will make the situation worse and possibly create a loop repeating the accusation

- Do have spares on hand for the items that get misplaced regularly to deescalate the situation when you "find" the missing object
- Don't ask the "why" questions. This is not rooted in reality and that may make her defensive
- Do use calm, reassuring statements that do not contradict the delusion such as, "We found your glasses," "You are safe now," or "I love you."
- Don't get angry or irritated
- Do give her a hug after she has calmed down

Crying or Laughing Sprees

Crying or laughing sprees usually occur in people in the moderate or early severe stages of dementia. Some people will alternate between laughing and crying off and on for hours.

Crying or laughing sprees happen because there is either an immediate need not being met or a chronic one. Doctors sometimes call it "emotional incontinence." These sprees can go on for hours.

With the immediate need, she may be releasing an emotion she cannot express any other way. Anything can trigger the event, from something specific, like too much noise, the lighting in the room being too dark or too bright or being laughed at by others. The issue could be larger like missing a deceased loved one, reliving a trauma, loneliness, boredom, or pain. It could also be they are self-aware enough to understand that something is not quite right, but they can't pinpoint the problem and are grieving the loss.

The two most common causes of the sprees are clinical depression and Pseudobulbar Affect (PBA). Folks with dementia are more prone to clinical depression than the rest of the population. PBA is a brain disorder caused by Alzheimer's and other kinds of brain injuries, such as concussions or strokes, that can affect the way the brain regulates emotion.[53]

When a crying or laughing spree takes place, try one of these suggestions:

- Be sympathetic. Try saying "You sound so unhappy. Can I help?" Never ask what's wrong, when she gets to this point, she may not be able to tell you what the issue is, and it may make the situation worse
- Be affectionate. Give her hugs or pat her on the shoulder or gentle rubs on the arm, etc. Reinforce the hugs or pats by saying things like, "You're safe," "It's okay," or "Everything is all right."
- Wrap her in a warm blanket
- Rub lotion onto her hands and arms

- Interrupt the behavior. Walk out of the room and come back with a warm drink or something to eat that will redirect the behavior. Try substituting something that will keep her busy and feeling useful, like giving her a baby doll or stuffed animal to hold, a fidget quilt, or batting a balloon, or blowing bubbles, or watching old slapstick movies, or finger painting, or setting the table
- If she went to church, offer to pray with her about "it." Even if you don't know what "it" is. Whether you are religious or not, sometimes something as simple as a prayer can calm the situation down
- Alert her doctor to the behavior. It is important to watch for symptoms of other types of depression, but it could also be PBA which is underdiagnosed in patients with Alzheimer's Disease. The unfortunate part is both require medication at a time in her life when less medication is better to prevent side effects. Depending on the severity of the crying, getting it treated may make life more enjoyable for everyone concerned

Every person with dementia will react differently, so these suggestions may or may not work for your situation.

It is okay not to be able to solve the problem. When someone cries, especially small children, we are hard wired to rush in and fix it. You can't always fix the crying sprees of someone with Alzheimer's. That's all right. The same goes for laughing sprees. Keep in mind that if you have been reassuring and addressed any medical problems, it is all that you can do.

Agitation — When the emotional volcano erupts

Agitation may develop in some people with dementia, and some people with dementia will naturally be highly anxious. It usually appears in the moderate stage of dementia. You may notice repetitive actions or fidgety behavior. She may fold then refold the newspaper or a shirt or rearrange knickknacks in the living room or rummage through the junk drawer. Most of the time she will remain calm and keep busy. Sometimes she may fly off the handle in a way that is out of sync with the situation at hand. Sometimes agitation will lead to an emotional eruption.

You may also notice behaviors like pacing, rummaging through the closet, swearing, screaming, and even aggression. It may also increase late in the day with Sundowning.

A number of things can lead to agitations:

- Hunger
- Exhaustion or sleep loss
- Dehydration
- Too much caffeine, sugar, or junk food.

- Adverse reaction to medication
- Stress caused from changes to the living environment, for example too many visitors, too much noise, a new caregiver, or a disruption in routine
- Feeling pressured in any way like being rushed
- Boredom, either from being left alone too long, or not having a constructive activity
- A change in schedule such as a late meal
- Her caregiver is in another room and she can't see them
- A psychiatric issue, such as being paranoid, angry, or scared. It might also occur when they are hallucinating or holding false beliefs
- A physical problem, such as an infection or a new or worsening chronic disease or pain. A sign it is pain: her behavior is completely different today from yesterday

When an episode of agitation erupts, stay calm. If this is a new or sudden behavior, get her in for a medical exam to rule out a physical cause.

- Avoid sudden movements, these can make her feel threatened
- Do not try to restrain her
- Do not respond to her in the same way—it will increase her agitation
- Don't scold or criticize her, it is important that you both get back to calm
- Do tell her she is all right
- Assure her you are there for her and that there is nothing to worry about
- Between each reassuring phrase, breathe in deeply through your nose and out through your mouth, she will copy your behavior

In instances when she is screaming or yelling and will not calm down, scream with her and urge her to scream it all out. Agree with everything she says. When you are in agreement, you can slowly calm the situation by taking deep breaths and breathing out. She will mirror your behavior and calm down with you.

Once the episode is over, try the following to avoid more agitated responses:

- If she is in a large room, move her to a smaller room. Smaller spaces feel safer to someone with dementia
- Reinforce routine; predictability feels safe and can ward off meltdowns
- In addition to routine, keep your living environment calm. Keep noise levels down including radio, television, computers, gaming consoles, and mobile devices
- Keep the lighting bright, but soft, nothing should cause glare; this includes closing window shades to block outside glare. Window shades should be

cordless to prevent accidents (See *Preparing Your Living Environment for Your Loved One*, page 71)

- Avoid activities that will cause her frustration. Choose activities where she can celebrate simple successes:
    - Setting the table
    - Consider activities like simple art projects such as pages for her memory book or finger painting
    - Listening to music
    - Singing
    - Going for a drive in the car
    - Making something or helping to make something like cookies or salad
    - Wrapping a present (even if there isn't a gift inside)
    - Wrap her in a warmed or weighted blanket to give her a feeling of safety
- Give yourself extra time for any challenging events like leaving for doctor's appointments. If she feels rushed, she may become agitated

Aggression

When your loved one acts hostile or with violence, such as lashing out verbally or physically, it indicates a change in brain chemistry and change in environmental factors, such as how they feel they are being treated. This usually occurs in the moderate stage of dementia. When an aggressive incident takes place, it is both upsetting and possibly dangerous for the caregivers.

The signs to watch for leading up to aggressive behavior are:[54]

- An underlying illness or physical issue
- A situation which makes her feel insecure or uncomfortable
- Personality shifts from mental changes, such as paranoia, anger, or fear
- Loss of inhibition and social boundaries
- A yet-to-be identified cause

Her anger is usually directed at the person who is helping her at the time, but it can also be directed toward other household members, pets, or objects. Sometimes the aggression can make her appear ungrateful, rude, or even mean. *This is a symptom of dementia.*

It is important you understand that the aggressive behavior is telling you something is wrong, and she can't tell you what it is anymore. Because she can't express her true feelings, which might be discomfort, frustration, anger, feeling out of control, or even fear, she physically expresses her feelings through behavior or acting out.

Another example: my sister took my father on an outing in February. He put on his coat but could not manage the zipper with his gloves on. My sister took the two ends of his coat out of his hands without asking his permission. When the zipper reached the halfway mark, my father's gloved fist connected with her face giving her a shiner.

Remember your loved one cannot change what is happening to her brain. **You** will have to change. Your biggest challenge is learning not to take it personally, not to respond in kind by raising your voice, not to act more forcefully, and not to threaten her. You may escalate the aggression. *People with dementia can still read body language and will respond in kind.*

<u>When you are faced with an aggressive response, here are some steps to try</u>:

<u>Take a step back from her, giving her space</u>. This will save you from bobbing or weaving if she swings or kicks.

<u>Stop doing whatever caused the outburst</u>. Whether it was trying to help her dress, take medication, or bathe, give her space. You both may need a moment to calm down. You can always try again later when everyone is less stressed.

<u>Stay calm and smile</u> even if you feel like whipping her with a towel. It must be a genuine smile, not a plastered-on smile. Ever fantasize about winning an Oscar? This is where your acting skills will come into play. Take a deep breath. Staying calm and smiling won't feel natural, but it will play better than escalating the situation and will help you both regain control.

<u>Talk to her in a gentle and respectful voice</u>. Speak calmly and slowly. Let her know you are sorry you upset her. Assure her everything is all right. Ask her if there is anything you can do to help.

It takes longer for a confused mind to calm down from agitation.

<u>*Whatever you do, do not repeat what you did to cause the outburst*</u>.

Quick Tip: Never act like you're in a hurry. One of the first instigators of agitation and aggression is you rushing to get to another task.

If none of this works, try one of these suggestions:
- Stepping out of the room for a little while so you can both calm down
- Suggest an alternate activity she enjoys like watching fish swim, eating ice cream, petting a stuffed toy, playing cards, or listening to a story. Chose her favorite activity
- Depending on her stage of dementia, walk out of the room, change your outfit, put your hair up, or put on a hat, and walk back in as a "new person" here to help her

Coping with Your Emotions after an Outburst

When you are coping with your own emotions after an outburst, don't be surprised if she doesn't remember the episode and behaves as if nothing ever happened. It is not a scam to manipulate you. Her brain is turning into Swiss cheese. *IT'S. THE. DISEASE.*

It is natural for you to feel hurt. You want to throw it back in her face. However, you are only hurting yourself by expressing your resentment to her later. She may mirror the same attitude back at you or retaliate in self-defense. Or worse yet, you will affect your own well-being by keeping your emotions tightly locked up inside you.

It's far better to have other outlets to express your emotions so that it doesn't hurt your health.

- Go for a short, fast-paced walk
- Punch your pillows
- Curse the heavens in private
- Go into your room and cry
- Have a couple of friends available by phone
- Use a Velcro bullseye and Velcro covered whiffle balls in your bedroom for target practice, that way you can throw something without causing damage
- Steal a page from my playbook and write in a journal or use laughter

Brené Brown, PhD, in her book, *Rising Strong, How the Ability to Reset Transforms the Way We Live, Love, Parent and Lead*, offers us the Tactical Breathing method, also known as Square Breathing and Box Breathing. It is a simple technique used to calm your heart rate and boost your ability to think clearly. It will help interrupt the intense fight-flight-or-freeze response after an unexpected encounter with your loved one and can be used as part of a meditation practice to improve your overall health. Breathing exercises initiate the rest-and-digest response, relaxing muscles.

Step 1: Breathe in through your nose for four seconds.
Step 2: Hold your breath for four seconds.
Step 3: Exhale through your mouth for four seconds.
Step 4: Hold your breath for four seconds.

Repeat until you relax.
You may experience a euphoric, tingling sensation if you do this for ten minutes or longer.

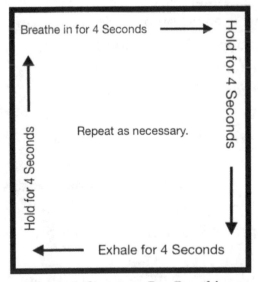

Figure 1, Square or Box Breathing

If you have difficulties falling asleep after an event, in addition to Box Breathing there is another breathing technique which may work, once you are in bed:

- Breathe in through your nose for four seconds
- Hold your breath for seven seconds
- Breathe out for eight seconds
- Repeat until you fall asleep

Choose something healthy; because neither drugs—not prescribed by your doctor, nor alcohol will help either of you in the end.

The Meltdown Trigger List

To reduce additional causes for aggression and other behaviors, check for the following:

What is her body language saying? Is she raising her voice, or is her voice shaking? Is her face red? Are her hands shaking? Has she traveled recently? Is she exhausted or sick? Has she started a new medication?

Drug interactions and side effects can cause new or different behaviors or worsening of symptoms, as can underlying health issues. Be sure to tell her doctor about dangerous behavior, in case it has been triggered by chronic pain, depression, delirium, infection, or other conditions which may be treated with medications.

> **The Meltdown Trigger List:**
> - Spreadsheet or note pad
> - Date, day of week and time
> - Where the event took place
> - A description of the physical surroundings with activities
> - Identify common event
> - Distraction techniques that work

Is there a new person or pet in the environment?

Are you doing something outside of her normal routine? Routine is the cornerstone of a stable living environment. Make sure you create safe and predictable surroundings and reinforce routine. Routine may help reduce agitation and aggression.

If the behavior continues, make notes listing what is occurring in your environment at the time of the outburst.[55] Medical professionals refer to this as chart notes.

Jot down the following (See template in *Appendix C* page 214):

- *What is the date?* Is it a holiday? Is it a family celebration?
- *What day of the week?* Is it only on Tuesdays?
- *What time of day is it?* Does the incident recur around the same time for each event?
- *Where did the event take place?* The living room? The bathroom? A restaurant? At church? A movie theater? A grocery store?
- *What are the weather conditions outside?* Sunny, calm, windy, snowing, raining, thunder, etc.

- *What is the temperature where the event took place?* Example: is it hot, warm, or cold? If you want to be more specific, 85 degrees Fahrenheit or 30 degrees Celsius.

- *What is the lighting like?* Are the lights on in the house? Is it dark? Are there candles burning? Are the shades drawn? Are there shadows being cast on the floor?

- *What type of activities are taking place?* Are you watching television, playing video games? Are children playing? Are you preparing a meal? Do you have company? Is there a crowd of people? Is anyone arguing?

- *What types of smells are present?* Coffee? Spaghetti-O's? Detergent? Household cleaners? Cigarette smoke? Scented candle? Urine?

- *What is the volume inside the house?* Is it quiet? Is there street noise? Sirens? Children playing? Dogs barking? Dishes being washed? Loud music? Multiple text pings? Loud video games?

If you keep your list up for three or more events, you will see a pattern develop. From there you can tailor possible solutions to prevent or reduce a repeat outburst. For example, does it always happen around dinner time? Did she used to prepare the family meal? Perhaps she feels like she should be doing something but does not know what to do. Give her a chore equal to her level of dementia like setting the table for dinner or dusting the furniture.

Here is an example of a meltdown log for Anita, whose challenging behavior is walking around the house banging the TV remote against the furniture and shouting when it is taken away.

Look for the common activity in each event	Event 1	Event 2	Event 3
Date, Day, Time	May 3rd, Tuesday, 3:35 p.m.	May 6th, Friday, 4:07 p.m.	May 8th, Sunday, 3:54 p.m.
Location	Family room	Throughout the house	Dining room and kitchen

Descriptions of physical surrounding with activities	It is bright and sunny, but cool outside. The TV is on, the window shades are up, the kids are home from school, dinner is in the oven and I am setting the dinner table.	Dark and raining outside. Shades are down. Dinner is cooking in the crockpot. Kids have friends over. The kids are playing music and talking in the family room.	Preparing meal early to go out to a movie with the family. Kids are helping. Bright sunny, warm spring day. Windows are open.

The common event for Anita, a former homemaker, begins with banging the remote in the mid-afternoon each day. When we look at what her family is doing, we see there is a lot of noise and activity in the house. She is Sundowning and seems to be confused. Her mind could be saying to her, "I know I should be doing something, but I don't know what it is" or "I need to get the house clean before dinner." Whatever she is thinking, the fix for this issue is to redirect her with an activity that she enjoys. In this example:

- Try substituting a cleaning rag for the remote. She may be confused about what to do with the rag. With her permission, gently remove the remote from her hand. Give her the rag and guide her hand in the motions for cleaning until she takes over.

- Perhaps a family member could take her for a walk, especially if she is pacing. It will give her time to socialize. Exercise can dissipate some of the energy that is built up from Sundowning and make her tired when it comes time to go to bed. Make sure the exercise is at least four hours before she goes to bed or she will be to wound up to sleep.

- Give her a "busy apron" to occupy her hands and her mind or a box of trinkets she can sort.

- Give her a photo album or scrapbook or her memory book with her story in it.

- There are also puzzles designed for people with dementia that have large pieces and simple patterns.

Give her an activity so she feels useful. If she cannot calm down, move her to a quiet part of the house and play soothing music, her favorite audio book, or her favorite television program.

Complete the Meltdown Trigger List so you can share it with family and friends:

Identify common event(s)	Kids are home, noise and activity: meal preparation	Kids are home, noise and activity: meal preparation	Kids are home, noise and activity: meal preparation
Distraction techniques that work	1. Replacing remote with cleaning rag 2. Setting the table 3. Walking to park and back with supervision while meal is prepared	4. Move Anita to her bedroom to listen to music	

The trigger list will also be effective with spotting other triggering events that could cause unwanted behaviors. Keeping a list of the things that triggered her aggressive behavior will help you avoid them. Make sure the rest of the family knows what the triggers are, so they don't end up with an unexpected black eye or worse.

You can do everything right and still trigger aggression in a confused mind that imagines a wrongdoing, or is afraid.

Medications are sometimes used to control aggressive behavior. Be sure to discuss with her doctor or pharmacist the benefits versus the risks of using drugs such as anti-anxiety, anti-depressants, or anti-psychotics. These drugs increase the risk of both stroke and sudden death. Because every person with A.D. reacts differently, they should be assessed based on their personal needs. In addition, current medical practices are changing. The medical field is reducing or eliminating the use of these drugs with Alzheimer's patients.

The bottom line is the least amount of medications are the best amount to reduce the possibility of side effects or adverse reactions.[56]

Long Term Coping Strategies for Aggressive Behavior

It is crushing and not uncommon for you to feel like you are living with a stranger. Especially if it is someone who has never behaved violently toward you before. This sort of aggressive behavior can be very isolating. You are not alone in that feeling. Contact a local support group or an online support network for the positive support you need. There is nothing wrong with asking for emotional support. It can be lifesaving. If you are caring for a spouse, visit the Well Spouse Association at www.wellspouse.org. See the *Resources* section for a list of additional online support, page 215.

Tendencies toward aggression often worsen over time. If you are ever in a situation where you do not feel safe, it may be time to consider the outside placement of your loved one in a memory care facility. It is often the case when a smaller partner cares for a much larger spouse who lashes out. No matter your size or strength, you are never too big to get outside help.

Consider asking your doctor, a local support group, the local chapter of the Alzheimer's Association, or any other available resource for tips on dealing with aggression and dementia. Also try contacting your local area agency on aging, these are state and federally funded organizations whose names vary from state to state. Start your search through the Association of Area Agencies on Aging, their website is: www.n4a.org. Otherwise, if you search the internet for "senior citizens" or "older adults" or "area agency on aging" you will usually find the listing. Your area's agency can help with locating available memory care facilities. They can also help you with other resources from legal assistance, respite care, in-home caregivers and home-based training programs for dementia caregivers.

One thing to consider, space is usually available for private pay patients such as those with long-term care insurance, but space is often limited for those on public support. You may have to wait up to a year or more for space to become available.

From Sexual Inhibitions to Sexual Aggression

We are human. Sexuality is a normal part of life no matter what your age, whether you have dementia or not. The person with dementia has the same urges as the rest of us but loses control of the mechanics which keep those urges in check or helps them differentiate what is appropriate and what isn't.

Sometimes they take off their clothes and wander around in a state of undress, sometimes they are overtly flirtatious, and sometimes they make unwanted advances. The behavior is more common among men than women.

Here is a list of the most common behaviors from the most frequent to the least:
- Making inappropriate comments
- Touching themselves or others
- Fondling themselves or others
- Undressing in public
- Making sexual advances
- Masturbating in public

The last three items happen in only ten percent of folks with dementia and usually as their dementia progresses farther along.[57]

Undressing in public happens when they are too warm, the clothing they are wearing is uncomfortable or itchy, they need to use the bathroom, they are having a delusion, they are bored or sexually aroused.

When naked happens, remain calm. She isn't trying to embarrass you. It is simply the way dementia works. When you remain low key, so will she. Simply remind her, "We don't do that here," or "Why don't we find a shirt or pants you like better. If you are in a public place, such as a restaurant, simply cover her and escort her to the bathroom for a little more privacy. A shawl works great as a quick cover.

Choose clothes and undergarments that are soft and don't have seams. Use pants or sweats that pull up. Choose tops that are pull over or fasten in the back. By simply changing the type of clothing they are wearing it can eliminate the issues. If it becomes a persistent issue, you can find Alzheimer Clothing (see *Personal Care*, page 116) that has special closures in the back so they cannot get out of it easily. Keep a spare set in your "Mom travel bag" (Earthquake preparedness kit). However, if they have to urinate frequently, this may create more work for you. (See *Emergency Preparedness*, page 40)

Try distracting her with an Alzheimer's "busy apron." The apron provides sensory stimulation by using a variety of activities and trinkets to touch. Some have zippers, cloth with different textures, buttons, ribbons, dangling keys, visual patterns, and are designed to engage her mind and fingers. It works for all stages of dementia. They are also a good tool for someone who fidgets obsessively. Busy aprons are available online.

While rare, aimless masturbation can sometimes occur in public. It can be very upsetting for you to witness. Keep in mind this is a result of a damaged brain. Do not overreact. Simply lead him to his room or the bathroom. Distract him by giving him something to keep busy with, such as a box of washers to sort or other items that will appeal to him. If he masturbates in front of children, the children are more likely to remember your reaction than what Grandpa Joe was doing. This type of masturbation can be caused by urinary tract infections, itching, or general discomfort. When this happens check with his physician for infection.

In some instances, a father may make inappropriate gestures toward their daughters. Generally speaking, it is not incestuous behavior. It usually means he has mistaken his daughter for his wife at the same age because he is not able to recognize familiar people as they are now.

When this happens, gently redirect him, then take a moment for yourself to recover. It can escalate.

To manage inappropriate behavior when it happens try the following:

- Stay calm and be patient
- In a firm but gentle voice, tell him what he is doing is inappropriate

- Match your body language to your words. Frown at him and shake your head. Remember he can still read body language
- Maintain firm and consistent boundaries. Don't encourage inappropriate behavior by sending mixed signals, like letting it happen one time then reacting negatively the next. Be consistent and be firm. Say things like "Stop that right now," or "No, I don't like that."
- Distract him or redirect him to a positive activity
    - Distraction: offer a snack, turn on the TV or ask an unrelated question
    - Redirection: Go for a walk or provide him with a favorite activity
- Move him to another location. This removes him from whatever triggered the behavior. Guide him to his bedroom or a quiet place if you are in a public area
- If none of the above works, raise your voice and firmly say "No" so that others in the area can hear you if you need help. Grab his hands and put them back in his lap. Look him in the eye, shake your head, frown at him, and let him know this is not acceptable. Raising your voice should shock him enough to redirect him

Here is an example from my own life to give you an idea.

My father and I sat in the waiting room of his Primary Care Physician's (PCP) office. About 25 other patients sat waiting, spread out through a waiting room which could seat 50 patients. Surveillance cameras poked through the ceiling tiles throughout the room.

My father's name was called. We stood up. He bowed to me and waved me to go ahead of him. When I reached the center of the room, a searing pain shot through my right butt cheek. I screamed. The room fell silent. My father let go.

Up to that point in my life, my father had never been inappropriate with me.

My body tensed. Adrenaline flooded my veins. I looked for an empty chair so I could beat him to death.

In my head I could hear one of my friend's voice reminding me to reframe.

Be calm, reframe. This is not my father; this is the disease.

I took a deep breath and looked around the room at the occupants. The mouth of every woman in the room hung open.

I took another deep breath and released it. I asked him, "Do you know I am your daughter?"

He leaned toward me and said, "*Yes,*" with a leer in his voice that sounded like a sex predator and nothing like my father.

Ignoring the praying mantis crawling up my spine, I

> **Reframing** is a technique used in cognitive behavioral therapy to create a different way of looking at a situation, person, or relationship by changing its meaning.

asked, "You know that's inappropriate?"

"No, it's not, you're my daughter."

I looked him in the eye and shook my head. Because I wasn't quite calm it came out in a verbal lash. "It's not appropriate behavior."

The Medical Assistant (MA) was too young and too shocked to say anything to my father's male Primary Care Provider (PCP), so the PCP could reinforce that it was not appropriate behavior. Remember people of a certain generation listen only to authority figures and men respond more appropriately to other men.

The PCP thought I was joking when I mentioned *the event*. Because the behavior was so uncharacteristic of my father, the doctor joked with my father about it.

When we returned to the car, I reminded my father the incident was recorded on the security cameras. His head hung and his shoulders dropped. He apologized for his behavior.

At this point in time my father was still able to understand the consequences of some of his actions. We talked about it later as a family—my husband, my father, and me. We discussed what my father would accept to redirect himself if he was behaving inappropriately with others. The lesson for me besides not going to prison for murder—this outcome would not have been possible without reframing.

Gun Safety

The ability to safely operate a motor vehicle involves memory, good judgement, and physical ability. These are the same criteria that should be used to assess a person with dementia's ability to possess firearms.[58] According to the Veterans Administration 40 percent of veterans with dementia own firearms. Alzheimer's changes everything including increasingly poor judgement and poor decision making.

For those who have hunted all their lives, it will be most difficult on those who hunted with him or her. If necessary, have his or her doctor or your clergy explain to your loved one's friends that dementia has now made it too dangerous for him or her to hunt or handle a weapon safely.

> *Remove or disable all firearms in the house.* Your loved one may mistake you for an intruder in your own home. If you choose to disable your firearms, there is still the danger your loved one may restore the weapon for use.

In an ideal world, once a diagnosis for dementia is given, you would set a firearm retirement date, which would be similar to an advance directive, for your loved one to voluntarily give up his weapons at some future point. This advanced directive would establish a "gun trust." It outlines how the weapons will be handled once he becomes incapacitated or dies. The trust can designate how the weapons will be passed on to family members, etc. These trusts ease the way for him to live in a space without weapons, such as in a nursing home or assisted living environment.

If you do not have a gun trust and cannot agree on a voluntary retirement date, put a plan in place if your loved one will not part with weapons voluntarily. While not ideal, when it becomes time to remove the weapons, choose a time when he is not home to make a safe transfer. Coordinate with a reliable family member or friend. It's your choice to store them, pass them on to a trusted family member or friend, or dispose of them.

If you still have issues with your loved one regarding the removal of firearms from your living environment, contact the local police or sheriff's office. They may request a statement of diagnosis from your loved one's doctor before removing any weapons.

If your loved one asks where the weapon(s) went, you can say things like, "It's out being cleaned," or "Joe borrowed it to go hunting." Be sure his friends will back you up if he calls them to return any "borrowed" weapon(s).

Your safety and the safety of your family is more important than your loved one's need to possess a weapon once his judgement deteriorates.

Wandering

According to the Alzheimer's Association, six out of ten people with dementia will wander. Ninety-four percent of people who wander are found within 1.5 miles of where they disappeared. If not found within a 24-hour period, up to half will suffer serious injury or death.

In the chapter *To Drive or Not to Drive, That is The Question*, we discussed Silver Alerts, page 28, and what happens when your loved one leaves home on their own. The causes of wandering vary by stages of dementia, knowing what level of dementia your loved one has may help you plan how to reacquire your loved one once they wander. Here are some techniques for preventing wandering or what to do if they lose their way.

Causes of Wandering:
- Feeling disoriented
- Getting lost
- Feeling restless
- Fear for their safety
- Overwhelmed by noise or loud sounds
- Boredom
- Needing an activity
- Needing exercise
- Needing to use the toilet
- Feeling hungry or thirsty
- Hallucination
- Brain damage from dementia

Level of Dementia

Mild Dementia

With mild dementia, create a cuing aid, such as a card for his wallet (or her purse), with instructions for when he becomes lost. For example, the card could be as simple as "I am Lost. Call home 555-555-5555" (use your phone number). Or if he goes to the same place regularly like a restaurant because he used to have breakfast there with his friends, write on the card, "Ask the server to seat you at a table and wait there. Call home 555-555-5555. I will pick you up."

You may need to create more than one card to cover different scenarios depending on where he goes, like the doctor's office, grocery store, coffee shop, etc. Keep in mind, men are less likely to admit to being lost and may feel they need to keep it a secret.

Once he reaches the late stage of mild cognitive impairment, he will get lost more often, even when going to places he has visited many times. Being lost can create feelings of panic. Reassure him if he feels lost, disoriented, or abandoned, by letting him know he is safe. Do not correct his fears, it will only reinforce his feelings; instead, redirect him. For example, if you are at home, say something like, "We are spending the night here tonight." "You're safe, I'm here with you." "We'll go home in the morning after some shuteye." You may have to repeat the reassuring phrase several times. This gives him permission to relax, knowing he still has the option to go "home" in the morning.

Moderate Dementia

When he reaches the moderate stage, it will be important to get him a dementia medical alert bracelet. Opening the clasp requires two hands, making it very difficult for someone with dementia to remove it. The typical information on the bracelet includes his name, medical condition, for example Alzheimer's, and instructions to call your number or the number of a monitoring service.

At this point, it will also be important to make modifications to your home to discourage wandering. See *Preparing Your Living Environment for Your Loved One*, page 71.

During this stage of dementia, hide the car keys. A person with dementia doesn't know they can't drive anymore, and they don't have any understanding of time. They can drive for 8 hours and think only 30 minutes have elapsed. See *To Drive or Not to Drive, That is The Question*, page 24, for more information.

As a precaution, take a picture of him each morning after he is dressed for the day so if he does wander off, you have a current photo for law enforcement, and can tell them exactly what he was wearing.

There are also subscription monitoring services which supply jewelry or watches with GPS (global positioning system) or RFID (radio frequency identification) locators so that when he wanders you can locate him. Another option is GPS or RFID locators placed in his car, on his motorcycle, scooter, or other vehicles.

Wandering can increase when there is a change in routine, like moving to a new living space, living with new people, joining a day care program, travel, or any other change in his environment.

There are different levels of wandering. If he is wandering around the house picking up objects and putting them down and no one is getting hurt, let him do it.

Another form of wandering is constant agitated pacing; it can be taxing on your nerves. Your loved one may be expressing a need to get away or go home. It can be hard to manage. It may be that something is scaring him. This could be due to a hallucination or not understanding what he sees, hears, or smells. It may also be caused by the brain damage from dementia and is not something he can control, which can cause agitation.

If you can't stop him from wandering or pacing by reassuring him that he is safe or giving him a task to redirect his energy, you may need to change your tactics. Give him a safe space in your home or yard to wander around. Or go for a walk together during the day to exhaust him enough that when Sundowners sets in, he won't feel the need to elope.

| To elope means a person with dementia wandered off. |

If he is very active, ensure he is eating enough food and drinking enough liquids. If he is underfed or dehydrated, this will add to his confusion.

When my diabetic father could no longer drive, he elected to walk. Because he walked so much, his blood sugar control improved and occasionally caused low blood sugars. He was living on his own when my sister found him unconscious one evening. He stayed in the hospital for a week. When he came out of the coma, his Alzheimer's disease escalated to the moderate stage.

Because he lived alone, the hospital would not release him to our care, but sent him to an adult family home. He was too active for the staff and, when they weren't paying attention, he would leave the home and take a walk by himself.

This behavior combined with his anger for being held prisoner, when he considered himself healthy, escalated his "bad behavior" and caused him to be sent to a series of different care facilities, each with tighter security. Each facility added medications to control his behavior. Eventually he was on ten different medications for behavior control. The drug interactions caused hyperactivity and spiked his blood sugars. When he was sent to the last and most secure skilled nursing facility, he asked the staff if he could go for a walk outside. After reviewing his file and seeing the words "elopement risk," they said no. My younger sister and I would take turns visiting him daily and take him on walks, but it wasn't enough.

Because no one at the facility would take his needs into account, he took matters into his own hands. Even though he had moderate dementia, the skills from his former profession were still clear in his mind. He noticed an issue with the mounting screws of the three-foot by five-foot plate-glass windows in his room. When his roommate went to physical therapy, he partially closed the door to his room. He removed the screws, lifted the window out of its frame, climbed out the window in his pajamas and slippers, replaced the glass, and fitted the screws back into the frame.

The staff discovered he was gone one hour later, but none of their security cameras showed him escaping. They called the police. Thirty minutes later 9-1-1 received reports of an elderly man in slippers and pajamas walking against the traffic lights on the main highway three miles from the facility.

The police brought him back to the facility. When the staff asked him how he escaped, he proudly demonstrated their security flaw. Their maintenance staff discovered 30 percent of the facility's windows had the issue, which they repaired.

When he could no longer exit via the window, he staked out the main entrance and charmed the lady visitors. Then he would gallantly escort them safely to their cars after their visit and go for his walk. After two more escapes, the facility put an alarm band on his wrist that sounded the alarm each time he neared an exit door. Employing his natural charisma, he hugged his favorite nurse when she left for the evening. He saw her punch in the exit code and noticed the visitor code next to the alarm pad. The next day he snuck out one final time. On December 23rd the facility gave us five days to find another location for him to live. They were ready for him to leave. That's when he moved in with my husband and me.

Identify the Triggers for Wandering

If he is having frequent wandering episodes, ask yourself the following:
1. What is happening before the episode?
2. Can you identify a pattern leading up to the elopement?
3. Does it happen around the same time every day?
4. Does it happen when he was asked to do a specific task like bathing or changing his clothes?
5. Are there other people living in the home? How are they reacting to his wandering within the home?
6. What is the noise level in his living environment?

Use the Meltdown Trigger List on page 102 to document the patterns triggering wandering, too. Once you figure out what may be causing the wandering, you may be able to manage it more easily. If you can't identify the trigger, it may be the dementia driving the behavior and all you can do is redirect him or distract him.

Create an Elopement Recovery Plan

Create a plan before you experience "wandering man." Just because he hasn't done it yet, doesn't mean he won't. Once he wanders off, you will have the same gut-wrenching feeling as losing your child in a crowd. Here is a guideline adapted from the Alzheimer's Association wandering plan:

1. Create a list of friends and family you can call for help. Make sure you have them on your cell phone contact list. Have a written list available for anyone who cares for your loved one when you are not there.
2. Ask your friends, family, and neighbors to call if they see your loved one outside alone.
3. Have your daily photo of your loved one handy, along with a close-up photo and his updated medical information available.
4. Know the dangerous areas in your neighborhood, such as stairwells, thick foliage, ravines, bodies of water, tunnels, bus stops, bridges, and heavily trafficked roads.
5. Is he right-handed or left-handed? Those with dementia tend to wander in the direction of their dominant hand. This may help you narrow down the search.
6. Create a list of places your loved one may wander. This could be places where they once lived, locations of former employers, places of worship, stores, bowling alleys, their favorite bars, restaurants, or coffee shops.
7. Consider enrolling your loved one with dementia in a wandering response service.

If your loved one does wander off, limit your search time to 15 minutes and then call 9-1-1. They will want to know where and when he was last seen.

The Reframing Technique

Let's talk a bit more about reframing. It is the technique I used to get through very difficult situations. I am not a trained therapist, nor do I claim any medical training. This is in no way intended to replace the advice of a medical professional.

With that in mind, reframing is another way to look at a situation, reduce stress, and recognize there may be more than one way to react to the situation you are experiencing. Think of it like a movie camera. If the camera is only focused on a bawling actress's face—her eyes are puffy with mascara running down her cheeks, that is your perspective. What happens when the camera pans back and you see her boyfriend proposing to her? You see and experience the context differently.

If you've never used reframing techniques before, try these steps:

1. Stop what you are doing
2. Take a deep breath
3. Think about the situation you are struggling with
4. What are you feeling in this situation?
5. What have or did you notice about the event?
6. Can you shift your perspective to something more positive?

In the example from the sexual aggression section. My immediate reaction was the defense mechanism of fight-flight-or-freeze. Pumped full of adrenaline, my initial reaction was defending myself without thought of the consequences. By changing my perspective, and briefly pausing to consider what was happening, I recognized that it was not my father, but the disease taking over, I was able to take a few deep breaths and chose a safer method of dealing with the situation despite being angry and in pain. After we talked about the event as a family, I learned new ways to redirect my father when his behavior was inappropriate that I would have never considered prior to the event. Win-win.

Since laughter is the biggest reward, once you have mastered the techniques in this chapter reward yourself with a leg lamp, the Academy Award equivalent for dementia care. According to Darren McGavin's character in *A Christmas Story*, "*It's a major award.*" You've earned it. Tee hee.

Chapter 12: Personal Care

"Wrinkles merely indicate where smiles have been."
~Mark Twain

One of the ways we differentiate ourselves from others is through our personal appearance. During the progression of dementia simple things like dressing, brushing our teeth, and shaving become more difficult. Eventually your loved one might not remember what a comb or a toothbrush are, or how to use them. They may wear their shoes on the wrong feet or wear their clothes inside out or backwards. They may not know what clothing is appropriate to the weather. They may not even know they need to change their clothing.

Personal care for your loved one requires patience and love, dignity and respect. There will be awkward moments whether bathing, getting dressed, or toileting. Treat them like you would like to be treated. While they may not remember a lot of things, they do have emotional-related memory and will remember being mistreated. Don't assume they will easily forget if they've been embarrassed, made to feel sad, hurt, or are in pain.

The bonus is they also remember events associated the positive feelings. For example, if bathing is rewarded by getting lotion massaged into their feet or hands afterwards, they will most likely enjoy the process.

Modesty Garments for Bathing and Toileting

One of the reasons an A.D. sufferer might refuse to bathe is the embarrassment of being seen naked. The Honor Guard is a modesty garment that can be used to cover private parts during dressing and bathing. It can reduce bath time troubles related to modesty issues. Men's and women's garments are available from the Dignity Resource Council (DRC) for both wet and dry uses. They range in sizes from "small-preteen" to 2X.

For those of you who might be experiencing a financial burden, the DRC offers free and discounted garments through their Love Covers program. For more information visit their website www.dignityrc.org or call their office at 844-678-4698.

Other options:

- Wrap her in a bathrobe or towel and wash her underneath it
- Sew two towels together like a poncho and bathe her underneath it
- Cut a hole in the middle of a sheet and drape it over her. You get the idea

Adaptive Clothing

Dressing becomes more difficult as dementia progresses. Now is the time to think about clothing that will be easier for your loved one to dress independently and to remain independent for a little longer. Eventually, your loved one will no longer be able to stay focused long enough to help with her own dressing. There may come a time when you are chasing a naked family member down the hall because she became distracted like a three-year-old.

Specialized clothes are designed to help people with arthritis or who are in a wheelchair to folks with incontinence or dementia. The clothing uses snaps and Velcro, no ties, no buttons. Here are websites for two companies who specialize in adaptive clothing.

Silverts: www.silverts.com

Buck and Buck: www.buckandbuck.com

Bathing Schedule

With all things dementia, the three most important words are: routine, routine, routine. When you are developing your bathing plan, the first thing to consider is what their routine was before the dementia set in. Did they bathe in the morning or evening? Was it a bath or a shower? Was it hot or cold? What did they call it? If they grew up taking baths, don't use the word shower. Did they call it a spit bath, soaks? Did they grow up taking sponge baths as a child? Perhaps they just need soap, a washcloth, and a cup or bowl of water. Whatever they called it growing up, use that term. It will meet with less resistance.

Do they have any fears associated with bathing? When one or more parts of the brain are deteriorating, noises can cause fear because they're no longer familiar. Things like running water, the fan, a dog barking, or people talking can all trigger fearful responses, if they become overstimulated. Past fears can play a large part in triggering resistance to bathing. Did they nearly drown at some point or were they molested in a bathroom? Are they extremely modest and don't want you to look? Have they forgotten the steps involved in bathing? My father was terrified of getting water on his face because he thought he might drown. We used a washcloth to protect his face and an adjustable shower head.

If you can figure out anything that might be triggering the resistance beyond dementia, you might have an easier time getting them to bathe. Use the meltdown trigger list to keep track of the issues so you can identify the cause(s) of the resistance. (See *Distraction Techniques*, page 86 or refer to *Appendix C*, page 214.)

They can get cold very quickly, especially if they are afraid. Wrap them in warm towels, a warm blanket, or their bathrobe after warming it in the dryer for ten minutes.

The Bathroom

On to the bathroom itself. Take a look at the bathroom. Let's step inside their head for a moment, what do you see? How does it feel?

- Does the bathroom feel too spacious? Is it so big that it doesn't feel like you will get any privacy? Try using curtains or shower curtains to create smaller, more intimate spaces in the bathroom

- What about clutter? Too many items lying on the counter, on the floor, or even in the tub/shower area will all cause confusion. Can you store the overflow elsewhere or consolidate? This includes removing multiple bottles of soap or shampoo

- Is the room or floor cold? Would it be possible to add a radiant panel to the wall, so the room is warmer?

- What color are the floor tiles? Are they white? This is an opportunity to add psychological warmth replacing the tiles with warm red tones.[59] It will also make white tubs and toilets easier for your loved one to find. If you cannot afford to remodel your bathroom, using colored non-slip mats next to the toilet and tub will help orient your loved one. Avoid black, dark blue, and dark brown colors

- What about the lighting? With dimming eyesight, daylight lighting is the most soothing type for people with dementia. They need bright light to eliminate shadows and glare. This will help them navigate the bathroom more safely and independently. Can you add a dimmer switch to accommodate the differing needs of the household? Night lights can help guide them to the bathroom at night

- What color towels are you using? They might not be able to differentiate a white towel from the wall or they may think a dark towel is a hole. Choose towels in mid-range colors so they can find them

- Mirror, Mirror on the wall . . . cover mirrors before your loved one enters the bathroom. Dementia causes them to think the mirror is a window and that somebody is watching them. A window shade makes a great cover. Just pull it down before they enter the bathroom and no more mirror. If you can't put a shade over the mirror, wet paper towels will work in a pinch to cover the mirror for the time you are in the bathroom

- A bidet is much less intrusive for cleaning private parts than your hands, if you have the option of adding one. If you don't know how they work, look for videos on YouTube
- A sitz bath is also an option. It is a bath in which only the hips and buttocks are immersed in warm water. It can be done in a bathtub or in a sitz bath basin which will fit onto the top of the toilet. It can be purchased online in kits. The more expensive kits will contain a hose which can be attached to a faucet for easier filling. Do not use soap, shower gel, or bubble bath in a sitz basin, it may cause skin irritation. To prevent infections, you can add up to a tablespoon of the following home remedies:
  - Baking Soda
  - Epsom salt
  - Sea salt (non-iodized)
  - Witch hazel
  - Vinegar
- Visual Aids: As dementia progresses, their vision reduces to tunnel vision. Place any bathing related items where they will see them, like a rubber ducky, attractive towels, washcloths. Anything to communicate that this is where to bathe
- Remove or hide anything that looks clinical, like Depends or transfer belts. See *Bathroom Safety Revisited* below
- Cover chrome (because of glare) in the bath or shower
- Are cleaning supplies visible where they can be confused for soap or shampoo or hair spray? Put them where they cannot be seen

Bathroom Safety Revisited

When inspecting the bathroom, make sure it is free of safety hazards that could potentially cause injury.

Here are some things to consider:

1. Is the door a pocket door? If it does not have a doorknob, they will not be able to figure out how to open it.
2. Is the floor clear of clutter that could cause a fall? Even a scale can be a trip hazard.
3. Is the floor level and non-slippery? Is there a wax coating on the floor? If so, remove it.

4. Are there safety-rated grab bars next to the toilet or in the tub/shower area? If not install them. Towel bars will not prevent a person from falling.

5. Can she safely get up or sit down on the toilet? If not, consider a raised toilet seat. Commode liners are available to ensure urine and feces go into the toilet. Do her feet touch the floor when she sits on the raised seat? If not, consider adding a toilet stool similar to a Squatty Potty for stability.

6. Is the tub/shower floor nonslip? If not, install nonslip mats or stickers or decals.

7. Is the bathtub spout cushioned? If not, purchase a foam cover to help reduce injury from a fall. They are available in most medical supply stores and in retail baby departments.

8. Is the tub/shower large enough to hold a bath chair? A chair will help you bathe her safely. Measure your tub's interior and exterior width, and then go online to check bathing chair dimensions. The legs should be adjustable. One part of the chair should be outside the bathtub making it easier for her to transfer into the tub. There are bathing chairs available with drop arms, so if you are transferring someone in a wheelchair it will ease the transfer. Most shower chairs are white. If your walls are white or light colored, consider putting a colored towel on the seat to help her find it.

9. Do you have a walk-in bathtub? Will she understand how to use it? Will she stay in the tub long enough for it to fill? Will she attempt to climb out before it fully drains? Will she open the door to the tub while the tub is full? If not, consider using a standard tub. If one is not available, use a handheld shower head for bathing or have distraction techniques ready to help her stay in place, such as storytelling, singing, bathtub toys for play, warm towels to wrap her in, massage lotion into her hands, giver her a baby doll to wash and care for, and a reward after bath time is done.

10. Is she too heavy or too big for you to lift her into and out of the tub? There are devices such as a bath lift or a slider chair. They are not cheap and can cost as much as $3,000. However, they are less expensive than remodeling your home. In the long run they will pay for themselves because you will not have to pay a professional caregiver to come in and do the bathing for you.

11. Is the water temperature too hot? If so, change the setting on the water heater to 120 degrees Fahrenheit (49°C) or lower to prevent scalding. Please note that A.D. patients may not perceive temperature in the same way you do. What feels comfortable to you may be too hot or too cold for her. Have her check the comfort level of the water before getting into the bath. Her ability to feel temperature will diminish over time and she won't be able to tell you if

something is too hot or too cold. Watch her for changes in skin color such as skin flushing for too hot, or blue lips or shivering for too cold.

12. What kind of flush toilet do you have? She may not be able to use a two-flush system toilet. You may need to install a toilet tank with handle. If she has arthritis, this is a must.

13. What kind of faucet does your bathroom sink have? Consider getting a lever-style faucet or tap turners, especially if your loved one has arthritis.

14. Are the faucets clearly labeled for hot and cold? Are the labels correct?

For ideas on properly installing items like grab bars and other bathroom safety features, visit ADABathroom.com. http://www.adabathroom.com/index

The Bathing Routine

Once you've identified when she normally bathes, how she bathes, and removed anything that causes fear or confusion, then routine and patience become all powerful. Emphasis on patience. There is power in routine. Bathing should take place at the same time every day. For someone with dementia, routine equals safety, routine equals independence. Routine reduces fear. Routine. Have I said that enough times? There might be a quiz later.

Pay attention to your body language. People with dementia can still read body language and will respond in kind. If you are relaxed, she will be relaxed. So smile or sing a happy tune she likes to sing and make it part of the routine. Be encouraging.[60]

Get everything ready before she gets in the bathroom. If you have to leave for an item, she will too. Make sure the bathroom is warm. Have the towels, washcloths, bar or liquid soap, and shampoo ready. Depending on the generation the person was raised in, liquid soap may be unfamiliar and threatening. Remember to limit the items in the bathroom to only what you need. If you are using a bathrobe for bathing, use three bathrobes. One to begin with, one for the bath and a robe warm from the dryer that provides a spa feel after bathing. Anything that feels like a reward will be remembered as a positive experience.

When she is beyond the mild stages of dementia, do not ask her if she wants to take a bath. The answer will be "No" or "I've already bathed." Instead guide her into the bathroom like you're going somewhere else and stumble upon the beguiling bath. Say to her, "Wouldn't it would be a shame to waste the water?"[61]

There may come a time when daily bathing is not feasible, and she will only bathe once or twice a week. Remember no one ever died from missing a bath.

Bathing Hints

- Make sure the bathroom floor is dry

- Have a non-slip bathmat
- If she is capable of bathing independently, let her do so. The more she can do on her own, the longer it will preserve brain function
- Complete one bathing task at a time. Do not rush
- Use a hand-held shower head. Do not hand her the hand-held shower head once she has reached the moderate stage of dementia unless you, the floor, walls, and ceiling want to take a shower, too
- If she merely needs prompting, give her the illusion of control by handing her the soap and washcloth. You may need to start the process by gently guiding her hand until she starts on her own
- If she cannot bathe on her own, start with washing her hands or feet first to get her more comfortable with the process
- When she has difficulty bathing, reassure her by saying things like, "We will take it slowly," "Can I help you with . . .?" "I am here if you need help."
- If she is an elderly person, use a gentle touch, do not scrub. Her skin is paper thin and sensitive. When towel drying, pat the skin, do not rub
- If she is still mobile, use a shower seat in the tub to create a familiar feeling environment
- If she is not very mobile, check her for pressure sores, red spots on the skin that are created when she is in one position for too long. Alert her physician if you find any. If left untreated they can become infected or worse—gaping open wounds, consider using bedsore rescue cushions
- If she enjoys bubble baths, music, or pleasant fragrances, do it. Anything to create a positive feeling. If she takes a bubble bath, make sure she rinses off before getting out of the tub to reduce the risk of a fall
- Washing hair can sometimes be challenging. Have her hold a washcloth against her forehead to prevent getting shampoo and water in her eyes. Using baby shampoo sometimes helps too
- If you are bathing a man, have him lean back against a bath pillow and put a warm washcloth on his face like he is at the barber shop. The bonus is he won't be able to see what you are doing. This may also work well for a woman
- Use soft towels. You may need more than one depending on the person. For example, did she wrap her head in a towel after bathing? Or do towels get dropped in the bath water? Is she modest? She might need six, ten or even 12 towels
- Distract her by talking about her favorite subject, singing songs, or reciting favorite nursery rhymes together

- Have her bathe a baby doll while she is getting bathed. <u>Hint</u>: if an arm or a leg falls off the doll, put it back on the doll right away. Otherwise you will have to deal with her panicking that the baby needs to go to the hospital. Don't be surprised if she carries the doll around with her like it's a real child

- Bribery never hurts. What does she like? Ice cream? Cookies? Hot coffee? If she preferred alcohol, substitute warm apple juice in a shot glass or tumbler, or grape juice or sparkling water in a wine glass. There will come a point when she will not know the difference

- Create spa coupons, sign names of her friends or family members and put them in a box. Tell her you need help with gift wrapping a present for a friend. Have her gift wrap the box the day before. You will leave the present on her pillow to find the next morning. Yay, present. Don't forget to reuse the gift certificates. Wrap, open, use, repeat

- If you are caring for someone who was formerly a businessman or businesswoman, have them sign in like it's a spa. They will be more cooperative

- If there is more than one of you taking care of her, try playing good caregiver, bad caregiver. When she gets upset, with bath giver number 1 (BG #1), have bath giver number 2 (BG #2)—the good caregiver, come in. Have BG #2 say to BG #1, "What you're doing is not okay. Get out of here." BG #1 leaves the bathroom. Then the "good" caregiver gets to apologize for her being upset and can ask if she would like help. She is more likely to cooperate with the one who saved the day. See *Distraction Techniques*, page 86

For additional ideas, check out Teepa Snow's videos on YouTube "10 Ways to De-escalate a Crisis," or "Helping a Distressed Person with Dementia" to learn how to de-escalate.

Bathing Hint Don'ts

- Don't use a whirlpool bath or jacuzzi. The bubbles look like boiling water to a confused mind
- Don't leave her alone in the bathtub. It only takes 2" of water for a person to drown

If you are still having issues with getting her to bathe, let's use what they do in memory care facilities: if it is a situation that occurs regularly, use the Rule of Three.

1. Remind her the night before that she will be bathing tomorrow evening.
2. Remind her after breakfast that she will be bathing before bed.
3. Remind her after dinner that she is bathing before bed.

If she needs more reminders, write it on her wipe board if you are using one. (See *Memory Aids and the Family*, page 29, for additional strategies.)

Using regular reminders may reinforce the idea in her mind so it won't be a surprise, and there may be less resistance.

You can always suggest that a handsome gentleman will be coming over later and ask her if she wants to freshen up.

Toileting Schedule

One of the main reasons people with dementia have incontinence is because they can no longer find the bathroom. For example, when she wakes up in the middle of the night, she will be disoriented. If she sees two doors (the closet and her bedroom door) and see lights under one of the doors, she will choose the door with the light under it. When she opens the door, the hallway presents several more doors. Which one is the bathroom? She is likely to try each one until she can't hold it anymore. Or he simply walks out his bedroom door, turns left at the potted plant and pees.

Learning your loved one's natural rhythms are a start to prevent clean-ups behind doors one, two, and three.

Urinary Incontinence

Before we discuss how to establish a toileting schedule, let's face it, incontinence happens, but it is not inevitable. If your loved one has an accident or can't go on command, do not yell at her or shame her. She is not three years old. She cannot prevent it from happening again without your help. You missed the cues. When out of the house, keep spare clothes and supplies in your "mom travel bag" a.k.a your earthquake preparedness kit (See *Emergency Preparedness*, Page 40.)

When we were potty training, we were taught "go" and "don't go" cues. We were taught to recognize certain clues, which meant it was not appropriate to "go," such as in public places or in front of other people. If you are asking her to urinate into a bedpan in bed, she might not be able to go because she doesn't want to wet the bed. The same may be true of a commode next to the bed. It's not the bathroom so she *knows* she shouldn't "go" there. Or is she in the restroom but is uncomfortable with someone watching, which is a "don't go?" Then, when she's out of the restroom, she can't hold it anymore and has an accident. The "go" clues could be taking down one's underpants or sitting on a toilet seat or, for a man, unzipping his fly.[62]

Things to consider when setting up a toileting schedule are restricting fluids after dinner, but not during the day. Dehydration can cause other issues such as infections, delirium, or behavioral issues such as agitation. Get a waterproof mattress or waterproof pads for her bed. Set it up so she is used to having it in place before she ever needs it. Trip hazards are another concern. Falls happen, especially at night. Make sure there are no area rugs and her slippers are not floppy or have slick soles so she can make it to the bathroom safely. (See *Preparing Your Living Environment for Your Loved One*, page 71.)

In the early stages of dementia, she may not always remember where the bathroom is. Put cueing aids on the bathroom door. For example, a picture of an outhouse. Leaving the light on in the bathroom with the door open at night will help her to remain independent longer. (See *Memory Aids and the Family*, page 29 for more ideas.)

Consider how she was raised. We have all had experiences where we had to use a port-a-bush to relieve that "go" situation. Was she taught to pee outside as a child or into a can in her bedroom when she was young? When considering men, did he pee off the porch at home, in the yard or potted plants or on the side of the road when traveling? Does he consider every freeway exit an opportunity? Knowing triggers ahead of time will help you prevent inappropriate urination in a waste basket, or in the ficus tree in the living room, or in the closet.

Plan a regular schedule by making notes of when she is usually answering nature's call. For example, immediately after she wakes up, or an hour after she drinks a cup of coffee. Does putting her bare feet on the cold floor in the morning make her incontinent?

She will give you visual clues such as picking or pulling at her clothing or becoming restless. A general rule of thumb if she doesn't give you any visual clues is to "go" every two hours. Expect to have to get up for toileting at least once per night. The more signs you recognize the less you have to clean up. Additionally, the more quickly she is cleaned up after an accident, the less likely she is to develop a rash or infection.

There are levels of incontinence: if it is only a leakage and not fully emptying the bladder, such as when someone laughs, coughs, sneezes, or exerts themselves, then using a light incontinence pad should help. They are available for both men and women. This way they may be less likely to be afraid to go out in public.

When it becomes more than just leakage, modern day incontinence supplies look more like underwear and less like diapers. You may have less resistance from her if she doesn't feel like she's trapped into wearing diapers.

Adult incontinence products are single use only. Most products list the amount of urine they can contain without leakage. A healthy adult bladder can hold up to 16 ounces of urine.[63] A full bladder can empty anywhere from 8 to 10 ounces of urine.[64] Personal earthquakes (emergencies) happen. Make sure you have spare supplies with you in her personal earthquake bag for such emergencies. Speaking from experience, take half a pack with you. You never know what can happen when you are away from home. Be prepared and you'll be far less stressed and won't have to change plans on the fly.

While some who have dementia will lose bladder control in the late stages of the disease, not all patients do. Several of the causes of incontinence can be controlled. If control is becoming an issue for her and if her doctor or nurse blows off incontinence as inevitable, get a referral to a doctor or nurse who has experience treating incontinence.

If she is showing signs of needing to go to the bathroom every few minutes, discuss this with her physician. It could be the sign of a bladder infection, drug interaction, or other health issue preventing her from completely draining her bladder. If there is no medical reason behind the urge, it could her way of saying she needs for more attention from you or other family members.

Watch for levels of comfort/discomfort. She will change as the dementia progresses.

When cleaning the floor after an accident, pet stain and odor removers work well on human waste. It's not just for your dog anymore.

Quick Tip: If your loved one is having difficulty starting to "go," but does not have a bladder infection or other health issue, hand her a glass of water with a straw and have her blow bubbles.[65] You may have to demonstrate if she is having difficulties following verbal instruction. She will relax and "go." It operates using the same principal as deep breathing exercises. The relaxation occurs when breathing out, thus blowing bubbles. It sounds crazy, but it works for both genders.

Please note that if you burn your garbage, when disposing of adult incontinence products, place them in the trash. Do not burn them, they will release toxic gasses that may cause you or your family serious health issues.

Bowel Incontinence

Abrupt loss of bowel control—temporary or otherwise—could be the sign of an infection, eating foods that encourage bowel movements (including mistaking cough drops for hard candies), diarrhea, medications, intestinal neuropathy, irritable bowels, constipation, or impacted bowels, should be discussed with her doctor.

> Impacted bowels means the stool is so hard it gets stuck in the colon or rectum causing excruciating pain. If left untreated it can cause death.

We are all adults here. Things are going to happen that you won't ever see coming. If she had an overwhelming and frightening hallucination, she could soil herself. You might be taking off her pants before she sits down on the toilet and she may spray fecal matter everywhere. It is not being done on purpose. It happens. You need to know it can happen, so you are prepared to clean the walls, toilet, floor, towels, clothing, and possibly even yourself. It can even be caused by traveling and being off routine. Unless you've had a colonoscopy, you may not understand how much stool one person can hold in their body.

We broke a washing machine at a laundromat because of a particularly nasty episode of serial diarrhea while traveling in a rented motorhome. We ran the machine for 24 hours trying to keep up with the mess. The machine died. The problem didn't. Personal earthquakes happen. After that trip we carried anti-diarrheal medication in the earthquake kit.

When working on your toileting schedule, figure out when she usually moves her bowels and get her on the toilet at that time. Make sure she can sit comfortably on the toilet—without pain or balance issues—long enough to take care of business. Make sure her feet rest on the floor. If she is too short to touch the floor, use a stable foot stool. Make sure she has something to hang onto like a grab bar or the handles of a safety toilet seat. By grabbing onto something, it will encourage her to stay put long enough to get the job done if she is prone to restlessness. If you need further distractions, play soothing music or give her a something to do like sorting through "treasures" in a jewelry box or craft box. It could include photos, buttons, small toys, coins, swatches of textured fabric, polished rocks, a tiny flashlight, anything she can touch without injury. If she is at the stage where everything goes into her mouth, supply her with larger objects like her memory book to look through, a soft book, or some other distraction device. (See *Memory Aids and the Family*, page 29 for more ideas.)

There are several options available to help with clean-up or prevent spillage, such as liners that make sure the urine and feces go into the toilet bowl. These are especially useful if you use a raised toilet seat. There are adult disposable wipes available and skin cleansing products that will reduce odors and liquify the feces making it easier to clean. Remember to wash your hands and her hands often with warm water and soap. The infection you prevent now may eliminate potential hospital bills later, so will taking time outs (respite) for your own mental and physical health. When in doubt, use the breathing exercise in *Self-Care* on page 132 to lower your blood pressure or use the box breathing method in *Distraction Techniques* on page 86.

Grooming

To get the best long-term benefit from grooming, try to maintain the grooming routine your loved one established for herself prior to getting dementia. Allow her to use her favorite products. Familiarity equals routine. Using her favorite products will reduce the confusion and/or fear that change can cause. The less you change her routine the longer she will be able to take care of herself, making your job easier.

Shaving

For men in the early stages of dementia, he may only need gentle reminders to get him to shave. Once the disease progresses, he will need help. If he uses an electric razor, he may be able to use it by himself because it has a large handle and requires little dexterity. Using the electric razor, he may be able to shave himself much farther into the disease with minimal coaching. Once he is having difficulties, you may need to guide his hand to get him going. Does he use a pre-shave lotion before using the electric razor? If yes, you may need to guide him through applying it.

When it is time for you to take over the shaving with the electric razor, use gentle, but firm circular motions. If he is becoming anxious, have a second electric shaver available for him to hold. Turn the electric shaver he is holding on so that he connects the two activities—you are shaving him while he is holding the other shaver.

If he prefers razors, use a safety razor. Drape a towel across his chest, tucked up under his chin to catch the water. Use a warm, wet washcloth to wet his beard. Then apply the shaving cream. Shave in the direction the hair is growing in short strokes. Rinse the razor often. Be careful when shaving sensitive areas. When finished shaving, rinse his face with a fresh, warm washcloth and pat his skin dry. After shave is optional.

For women with dementia, shaving is optional. Once a woman is in the moderate stages of dementia it may not be worth the battle.

Hair Styling and Makeup

For men and women, once they have reached the point where they need help with their hair, it's time to consider short, simple haircuts. This will make it easier for them to remain somewhat independent a little bit longer. You may only have to remind them to comb their hair at first. Farther into the disease, you will need to guide their hand to get them started. Eventually you will need to take over their hair care for them.

Regarding makeup, once she's reached the moderate stage, just give her a little lip color.

When you are finished with grooming tell your loved one how wonderful he or she looks. Positive comments go a long way toward a good behavior day.

Nail Care and Foot Care

Normal aging can make it more difficult to take care of simple tasks like bending over and trimming toenails. When we add dementia to the mix, she may forget how to trim her fingernails or toenails. She may not even recognize clippers, scissors, or toenail trimmers. With some forms of dementia, balance and coordination may also become a problem. In addition, there are also common issues as we age, such as bunions or calluses which can cause pain, but she may not be able to tell you there is an issue.

Setting up a routine for nail and foot care is essential to preventing minor issues from becoming serious problems. If you choose to groom her feet, check for signs of skin irritation that might show problems with her shoes.

Toenails can thicken, requiring a special type of toenail trimmer, such as a heavy grade or medical-grade toenail trimmer. If you do not have the strength to cut her toenails or do not feel comfortable with foot care, take her to a podiatrist (foot doctor) who can manage the foot care for you. It is better to take care of her feet before a minor problem becomes a serious one. If personal finances allow, take her to a day spa every six weeks for a manicure, pedicure, and getting her hair done. She will feel wonderful and you will get some much-needed respite time.

Oral Hygiene

Beware that dazzling smile, it has teeth and may bite.

Brushing, flossing, and gargling are not without risk when working with someone with dementia. Taking care of your loved one's teeth, while challenging, can prevent pain from gum infections, cavities, and abscessed teeth. Pain is one of the leading triggers for agitation and violence in people with dementia. Sores in their mouths can lead to other problems including speeding up their mental decline.

People with A.D. and dementia have many eating challenges ahead of them, *including* not chewing well and choking on food, or inhaling food into their lungs and getting pneumonia—the leading cause of death among A.D. sufferers.[66] If they are experiencing dental pain or have ill-fitting dentures, they may refuse to eat. Keeping up on dental work is very important. However, having a dentist specifically trained to deal with dementia is also important. If a dentist or hygienist tells you they work with dementia patients all the time but will not let you be present during the cleaning, choose another dentist. Causing your loved one anxiety because unfamiliar people are "attacking her" is not worth the heart ache.

When working with the dentist or dental hygienist, provide them with a list of her medications. If they aren't already doing so, ask them to play soft music and speak slowly with a calm voice as they explain each step before they proceed with it.

Cleaning Teeth and Dentures

When brushing teeth, choose the right tool for the job. Choose a soft bristle toothbrush with a large handle, such as a child's toothbrush without the juvenile elements. Or add an adaptive foam handle such as those used for people with arthritis so when they begin to lose their fine motor skills, they will still be able to grip the toothbrush. An electric toothbrush has a large grip and some people will prefer it to a regular toothbrush.

In the early stages of dementia, she may simply forget to brush her teeth and need to be reminded.

In the moderate stage, she may find it too complicated without simple directions:

- Put the toothpaste on the toothbrush and set it in front of her. If she doesn't clue-in to the visual prompt . . .
- Walk her through each step. For example: "Pick up the toothbrush," "Put it in your mouth," "Brush the top teeth," "Now brush the bottom teeth" and so on.

If she still seems confused, she will be able to mimic what you do. It will relieve her fears seeing someone else demonstrate. So, jump right in and do your teeth at the same time. The best part is it will give you time for a little more YOU-time once she's in bed.

At some point, getting her to brush her teeth may become too exhausting for her and might only happen in the morning when she is not tired.

When it gets to the point where you will be brushing her teeth for her:

- Have her sit in a chair and tilt her head back
- You may find it easier to stand behind her to clean her teeth and gums
- Put a small amount of toothpaste on a soft bristle toothbrush or leave it dry
- If the toothbrush is unacceptable you can purchase sponge-tipped swabs filled with toothpaste. It is softer on the gums and swabbing may be more acceptable to her. They can be used after every meal
- Offer a small cup of water to rinse. It's okay if she swallows if you didn't use very much toothpaste
- While dental floss is recommended, it will become too much of a hassle. Try using floss picks

Even if she has given you permission to brush or floss, she may forget or change her mind and then bite you. Then you need to convince her to let go, all while you stay calm and suppress a scream.

Dentures present their own hazards. She should have her dentures in when she eats. If the dentures don't fit well, she will stop eating foods she cannot chew. Ill-fitting dentures can cause gum sores. The same is true if the denture adhesive is not applied correctly. This can cause poor nutrition or even constipation. If her dentures don't fit properly, take her to the dentist and get them fixed.

If she can no longer care for her dentures, for example forgetting to clean them or refusing to take them out, you will need to take over care to prevent gum sores from developing.

- Remove dentures for at least 4 hours every day
- Clean dentures daily

- Check for gum sores daily
- Learn to apply the denture adhesive for best fit

Quick tip: To gain her cooperation in removing her dentures, make it a fun experience, like:

- Reading together after lunch or dinner, then remove her dentures with dessert as a reward at the end like soft-served or softened ice cream
- If she is a creative person, perhaps sponge painting with stencils after she removes her dentures

Chose an activity that matches her skill level. If the activity is done every day, she may not remember to remove her dentures without prompting, but she will remember the happy feelings surrounding the routine.

When the dentures are not in her mouth, be sure to put them in the same place every time so they do not get lost. It is very common for denture wearers with dementia to hide their dentures overnight thinking they are saving them in a safe place. For example, you may have to spend some time searching until you find them. She won't remember she put them between two paper plates and duct-taped the plates together, then hid them in: the dryer, her underwear drawer, in a potted plant, in the fish tank, in the garbage can, etc. for safe keeping. Remember to breathe deeply and laugh about it at work later.

Schedule an appointment for her regular dental check-up at least once a year, or more often if she develops chronic issues.

Eye Care

Glasses, glasses, who's got the glasses? If your loved one wears glasses, be prepared to spend time searching for misplaced glasses. This will start in the mild cognitive impairment stage. Keep a previous pair or some readers handy in case the current glasses are so well hidden you can't find them. Also keep a copy of her prescription on hand in case her glasses are lost while traveling.

By the moderate stage of dementia, she may forget she even needs to wear them. Forgetting to wear glasses can cause two problems: first, it will affect her mobility and safety as she moves within her living space; and second, without her glasses she will have less visual stimulation, speeding up the progression of the disease.

Eye health is another important factor. Preventing or treating glaucoma and cataracts will prevent blindness. If possible, take her to an ophthalmologist (eye doctor), who specializes in dementia care, at least once a year.

Self-Care

Did you know that as a dementia caregiver you are holding your breath and causing your cortisol levels to rise? Cortisol is great if you are outrunning an angry mob with clubs and pitchforks, but not so great when you are banking it every day in your body for retirement. When we are stressed, we hold our breath—only using the top third of our lungs. It increases blood pressure, chances of heart attack, likelihood of diabetes, and chances of early death. [67]

If you use this simple breathing technique five times a day. Over the course of six months your cortisol levels will return to normal.

Follow these simple steps to reduce your daily stress:

1. Take a step back from whatever you are doing.
2. Take a deep breath in through your nose, fill your lungs until you feel it in your diaphragm (belly).
3. Gently purse your lips together and breathe out for 8 seconds.

   Repeat two more times.

Quick tip: Set the alarm on your cell phone so you don't forget to take time to breathe. Dementia caregivers are the most likely of all caregiving groups to put off self-care.

Chapter 13: What's for Dinner?

Former restaurant owner Cathy Russell created easy to prepare recipes for her parents when they began the journey of cognitive decline. They needed help with meal preparation while still remaining independent.

She now uses these recipes to teach non-cooking caregivers simple menu planning and meal preparation, paired with grocery lists for each week's menus, taking the guesswork out of shopping.

If you are feeding only two people, the leftovers can be refrigerated or frozen for another quick meal and reheated in the microwave or oven using microwave or oven safe dishes.

Safety note: hot from the oven glass dishes and hot ceramic dishes, when set in cool or cold spilled liquids like water, will explode and can cause injury.

Week One

Shopping List

1 six-pound package of boneless, skinless, chicken breasts

1 four-pound package of ground beef

1 small fully cooked ham

2 cans condensed Cream of Chicken soup

1 can condensed Tomato soup

1 small bag frozen mixed vegetables

1 16 oz. bag California Blend frozen vegetables

1 small bag frozen broccoli florets

1 envelope Knorr Pesto sauce or Creamy Pesto sauce mix

1 Onion

5 lb. bag potatoes

1 package penne pasta 8 to 16 oz.

1 package shredded cheddar cheese
1 package shredded parmesan cheese

Check the Pantry For

Olive oil
Dried onion flakes
Rice
Bisquick
Milk
Eggs
Bread
Canned greens beans

* * *

Pesto Chicken Pasta

Make ahead tip: Chicken breasts can be pre-cooked, cut up, and stored in one or two cup containers, then refrigerated for up to 3 days or frozen for later use to speed up food preparation time.

Preparation Time 50 minutes

Total time 1 hour 10 minutes

Equipment

1 cup liquid measure

1 cup dry measure

4 to 6-quart saucepan

4 to 6-quart heavy bottom pot or Dutch oven

Whisk

Wooden spoon or heat resistant spatula

Large strainer

Paring knife or meat thermometer

Medium mixing bowl

Small mixing bowl (microwave safe)

Recipe

8 oz. penne pasta (half of the package)

1 envelope Knorr Pesto Sauce Mix or Creamy Pesto Sauce

3/4 cup milk

1/4 cup olive oil

2 cups cooked, cubed, chicken (3/4 pound)

1 cup frozen broccoli florets

Shredded Parmesan cheese

Prepare chicken: Fill pot with 3 to 4 cups of water, add raw chicken. Bring water to a simmer. Put lid on pot and cook for 8 to 10 minutes. Make sure the chicken is cooked to 160°F (71°C), or no pink left inside when you run a paring knife through the thickest part. Juices from chicken should be clear. Place chicken in medium bowl to cool. Let cool for 10 minutes then cut into ½″ cubes. Set aside. Wash pot for use with pasta.

> Simmering water is just below boiling point. The water, when heated, will give off small, steady bubbles.

Cook the pasta according to package directions.

Meanwhile, in a large saucepan, whisk together pasta mix, milk, and oil. Bring to a boil. Reduce heat to medium-low; simmer, uncovered for 5 minutes. Cook frozen broccoli in the small bowl in microwave with 1 tablespoon water for 3 to 5 minutes. Add chicken and broccoli to saucepan; heat through. Drain pasta. Add to the sauce and toss to coat. Sprinkle with parmesan cheese.

Easy Chicken Pot Pie
Preparation Time 50 minutes
Total Time 1 hour 20 minutes
Equipment
1 cup dry measure
2 cup liquid measure
Heavy bottomed pan or Dutch oven
10″ deep dish pie pan
Spatula or wooden spoon
Dinner plate
Medium mixing bowl
Meat thermometer or paring knife
Aluminum foil
Recipe
1-2/3 cups frozen mixed vegetables, thawed

1 cup cubed, cooked chicken

1 can (10-3/4 oz.) condensed Cream of Chicken soup

1 cup Bisquick mix

1/2 cup milk

1 egg

Preheat oven to 400° F (204° C).

Prepare chicken: Fill pot with 3 to 4 cups of water, add raw chicken. Bring water to a simmer. Put lid on pot and cook for 8 to 10 minutes. Make sure the chicken is cooked to 160°F (71°C), or no pink left inside when you run a paring knife through the thickest part. Juices from chicken should be clear. Place chicken on a dinner plate and loosely tent with foil to cool. Let cool for 10 minutes then cut into ½" cubes. Set aside in bowl.

In greased 10-inch, deep dish pie pan, stir together vegetables, chicken, and soup.

In medium bowl, stir Bisquick, milk, and egg until blended. Spread over top of pie. Bake about 30 minutes.

Alternate crust option: frozen pie dough. Follow package instructions for thawing dough. After cooking 20 minutes cover edge of pie dough with aluminum foil for last ten minutes of baking to prevent crust from burning.

Meatloaf and Baked Potatoes
Preparation time 30 minutes
Total time 2 hours
<u>Equipment</u>
Fork
Large bowl
Loaf pan or 11" x 7" x 2" baking pan
<u>Recipe</u>
1-1/2 pounds ground beef

1 slice bread

1 egg

1/2 cup milk

1 tablespoon dried onion flakes

Preheat oven to 350° F (177° C). Scrub two medium potatoes, prick with a fork several times, and place in oven. Bake 350° F (177° C) for 1 hour and 30 minutes. Prepare meatloaf: in a large bowl, soak bread slice in milk. Add egg, ground beef, and onion flakes. Using hands mix all ingredients together. Pat into a loaf pan or shape into a loaf and place in a 11 x 7 x 2" pan. Bake 350° F (177° C) for 1 hour.

Serve with vegetable of your choice.

Shepherd's Pie
Preparation time 30 minutes
Total time 1 hour

Equipment

Large skillet	1 cup liquid measure
1-½ quart casserole or 10-inch, deep dish pie pan	Peeler
Potato masher, potato ricer or immersion blender	Paring knife
Stock pot	Wooden spoon or heat resistant spatula
	Can opener
½ teaspoon measure	
½ cup dry measure	

Recipe

1-pound ground beef	1/2 cup warm milk
1/2 teaspoon salt	1 beaten egg
1 can (15 oz.) green beans, drained	1/2 cup chopped onion
1 can (10 3/4 oz.) condensed tomato soup	Dash pepper
5 medium potatoes, cooked and drained	1 tablespoon butter or non-stick cooking spray to grease casserole or pie pan

Preheat oven to 350° F (177° C). Prepare potatoes: scrub and peel two medium potatoes. Cut potatoes in half, cut the halves into three even pieces. Put potatoes in stock pot. Fill pot with water to cover the potatoes. Bring pot to boil over medium-high heat. Boil potatoes without lid for 10 to 15 minutes or until a knife can be inserted into the potato without resistance. Drain water from pot. Cover pot with lid and set aside (off heat).

In large skillet, cook meat and onion over medium heat, breaking up meat as it cooks. Cook until meat is lightly browned, and onion is tender, 3 to 5 minutes. Add salt and pepper. Add drained beans and soup and mix together; pour into greased 1-½ quart casserole or 10-inch, deep dish pie pan. Mash potatoes while hot; add milk and egg, mix together. Season with salt and pepper. Spoon potatoes in mounds over casserole. Bake at 350° F (177° C) for 25 to 30 minutes.

Ham and Rice Bake

Preparation time 30 minutes

Total time 1 hour

Equipment

Large saucepan

Wooden spoon or heat resistant spatula

1-½ quart casserole dish

1 cup dry measure

Small bowl

Can opener

Recipe

1 can (10 3/4 oz.) condensed cream of chicken soup

1 cup shredded cheddar cheese, divided (Hint: (2) ½ cups of cheese)

1 16 oz. package California Blend frozen vegetables, thawed

1 cup cooked rice

1 cup cubed fully cooked ham

Preheat oven to 350°F (177°C). Prepare ham: cut fully cooked ham into ½" cubes. Put into small bowl. Set aside.

Cook rice according to package directions. (Hint: ½ cup uncooked rice will make 1 cup cooked rice.)

In a large saucepan, combine the soup and 1/2 cup of the cheese; cook over medium heat and stir until the cheese is melted. Stir in vegetables, rice, and ham. Transfer to a greased 1-½ quart casserole dish. Sprinkle with remaining cheese. Bake uncovered for 25 to 30 minutes.

Week Two

Week Two Shopping List

4 boneless pork chops

1 29 oz. can peach halves

1 15 oz. can black beans

1 15 oz. can corn

1 can condensed Cream of Celery soup

1 jar salsa

1 package taco seasoning

1 package flour tortillas

1 16 oz. package fresh sliced mushrooms

1 package (8 oz.) wide egg noodles

1 small bag frozen petite peas

1 package shredded Swiss cheese

1 package shredded Mozzarella cheese

1 package shredded cheddar cheese

1 box chicken broth or granules

1 box beef broth or granules

1 head lettuce

1 large tomato

Check Pantry For

Breadcrumbs
Corn Flake crumbs
Eggs
Grated parmesan cheese
French's Fried Onion Pieces
Dry ground mustard

Parmesan Pork Chops and Peaches
Preparation time 30 minutes
Total time 1 hour 15 minutes
Equipment
1-gallon resealable plastic bag
Small Bowl
Fork
1 tablespoon measure
1 teaspoon measure
¼ teaspoon measure
9" x 13" baking dish
Can opener

<u>Recipe</u>

1/2 cup bread or corn flake crumbs	2 tablespoons grated Parmesan cheese
1 teaspoon salt	1/4 teaspoon pepper
4 boneless pork chops	1 egg, beaten
1 1 lb. 13 oz. can peach halves, drained	brown sugar

Preheat oven to 425° F (218° C). Combine crumbs, parmesan cheese, salt, and pepper in a resealable plastic bag. Break egg put white and yolk into small bowl. Using a fork, stir the egg until yolk and white are combined. Dip pork chop in egg until chop is fully coated with egg. Put chop in resealable plastic bag with crumb mixture then shake. Place coated chops in a 9 x 13 x 2" baking dish and bake for 30 to 35 minutes (40 to 45 minutes for 1" thick chops.) During last 10 minutes of baking add drained peach halves and sprinkle with brown sugar.

Prepare boiled potatoes: scrub and peel 2 medium potatoes. Cut potatoes in half, cut the halves into three even pieces. Put potatoes in stock pot. Fill pot with water to cover the potatoes. Bring pot to boil over medium-high heat. Boil potatoes without lid for 10 to 15 minutes or until a knife can be inserted into the potato without resistance. Drain water from pot. Cover pot with lid and set aside (off heat).

Serve with boiled potatoes and vegetable of your choice.

Soft Chicken Tacos

Preparation time 30 minutes

Total time 45 minutes

<u>Equipment</u>

10" to 12" frying pan

Heat resistant spatula or tongs

1 tablespoon measure

Chef's knife (8 to 10" long)

Paring knife or serrated kitchen knife

Can opener

Meat thermometer

1 cup liquid measure

Dinner plate

Aluminum foil

<u>Recipe</u>

2 boneless, skinless chicken breasts, cubed   Flour tortillas

1 tablespoon vegetable oil

1 15 oz. can black beans, drained and rinsed

1 15 oz. can corn, drained

1 cup salsa

1 tablespoon taco seasoning

Shredded lettuce

Shredded cheddar cheese

Diced tomatoes

Sour cream

Cut raw chicken into ½" cubes. Heat oil in pan over medium-high heat for two minutes until oil is just smoking. Cook chicken in skillet for 6 minutes stirring frequently and then add the taco seasoning and mix so the chicken is well coated. Add the corn, black beans, and salsa to pan and heat through. Remove from heat.

While chicken mixture is cooling shred lettuce and dice tomatoes.

To shred lettuce by hand, wash lettuce thoroughly. Cut the head of lettuce in half through the core, then cut into quarters. Put a quarter section of the lettuce, flat side down, on the cutting board. Hold the chef's knife perpendicular to the wedge. Cut the wedge in 1/8- to ¼-inch thick shreds.

To dice a tomato, remove all stickers and wash it thoroughly. Cut it in half through the core using a very sharp paring knife or a serrated kitchen knife. Slice the tomato into ¼ to ½ inch thick slices. Stack a couple of slices together and cut into strips. Next cut the tomato strips into the same size dice. Set aside in a small bowl.

Put about 1/3 of a cup of filling in a 10" flour tortilla, top with cheese, tomato, lettuce and sour cream. Fold the tortilla up one third, fold in the two ends and fold over last third to wrap the tortilla.

Country Ham Casserole
Preparation time 30 minutes
Total time 1 hour 5 minutes
Equipment
Can opener
1 cup liquid measure
1 cup dry measure
½ cup dry measure
½ teaspoon measure
Stock pot or 3-quart saucepan
3-quart casserole dish
Wooden spoon or heat resistant spatula

Recipe

1 can (10 3/4 oz.) condensed Cream of Celery soup

3/4 cup milk

1/2 teaspoon dry mustard (optional)

1 package (8 oz.) wide egg noodles, cooked according to package directions, drained

2 cups cubed ham (about 1/4 lb.)

1 1/2 cups shredded Swiss cheese, divided (Hint: 1-1/4 cup and ¼ cup)

1 cup frozen green peas

French's Fried Onion Pieces

Preheat oven to 350°F (177°C). Prepare ham: cut fully cooked ham into ½" cubes. Put into small bowl. Set aside. Cook noodles according to package directions. Drain and set aside.

In a 3-quart casserole dish combine soup, milk, and mustard. Stir in noodles, ham, 1-1/4 cups Swiss cheese, and peas. Bake covered 30 minutes. Remove cover, top with remaining cheese and fried onion pieces. Bake an additional 5 minutes.

Mushroom Smothered Salisbury Steak

Preparation time 30 minutes

Total time 45 minutes

Equipment

Can opener

¼ teaspoon measure

1 tablespoon measure

1 cup liquid measure

Whisk

Small bowl

Large bowl

12" non-stick skillet

Cooking spray

Dinner plate

Aluminum foil

Recipe

1 can beef broth

3 tablespoons flour

1/2 cup picante sauce, divided

(Hint ¼ cup each)

3 tablespoons breadcrumbs

1 large egg

1/2 package (8 oz.) sliced mushrooms

12 ounces ground beef

Salt

Combine beef broth, flour, 1/8 teaspoon salt in a small bowl and stir with a whisk. Add 1/4 cup picante sauce, stir well and set aside. Combine beef, breadcrumbs, egg, and 1/4 cup picante sauce and 1/4 teaspoon salt in a large bowl. Divide meat mixture into four equal portions shaping into a ½-inch thick patty.

Coat large non-stick skillet with cooking spray. Heat skillet over medium heat. Add patties and cook 5 minutes on each side. Remove patties from pan, place on dinner plate and cover with aluminum foil to keep warm. Add mushrooms to the pan and sauté for 2 minutes or until browned. Add broth mixture to pan. Bring to a boil. Stirring constantly, cook 3 minutes or until slightly thick. Return patties to pan and cook until heated through.

Serve with mashed potatoes and vegetable of your choice.

Baked Mushroom Chicken

Preparation time 30 minutes

Total time 1 hour

<u>Equipment</u>

¼ cup dry measure

Cling wrap

Chef's knife

Meat pounder or heavy bottomed saucepan

Gallon-size resealable plastic bag

12" skillet

11" x 7" baking pan

Non-stick cooking spray

Spoon

Wooden spoon or heat resistant spatula

Tongs

<u>Recipe</u>

4 boneless skinless chicken breasts (about 1 pound)

1/4 cup all-purpose flour

3 tablespoons butter, divided (Hint: 2 tablespoons and 1 tablespoon)

1 cup sliced fresh mushrooms

1/2 cup chicken broth

1/4 teaspoon salt

1/8 teaspoon pepper

1/3 cup shredded Mozzarella cheese

1/3 cup grated Parmesan cheese

Preheat oven to 375° F (191°C). Spray 11″ x 7″ baking pan with cooking spray, set aside.

Flatten each chicken breast to ¼-inch thickness: lay chicken breast flat on cutting board, smooth side facing up. Place your hand flat on top of the chicken. Using the chef's knife, slice the chicken in half, horizontally. Place the cutlets, smooth side down on a large sheet of cling wrap on the cutting board. Place another sheet on top to prevent splatter. Using a meat pounder or a heavy bottomed saucepan, pound the cutlets until they are uniformly ¼″ thick.

Place flour in a resealable plastic bag; add chicken 2 pieces at a time. Seal bag and toss to coat (Hint: shake bag). Heat 2 tablespoons of butter in a large skillet over medium-high heat until bubbling, add chicken and cook about 2 minutes on each side. Transfer chicken to prepared 11″ x 7″ baking dish. In the same skillet, add remaining tablespoon of butter, add mushrooms. Sauté mushrooms until tender. Add the broth, salt, and pepper, and bring to a boil. Cook for 5 minutes or until liquid is reduced to about 1/2 cup. Spoon over chicken.

Put chicken in oven. Bake uncovered for 15 minutes or until chicken is no longer pink. Sprinkle with cheeses. Bake 5 minutes longer or until cheese is melted.

Serve with potatoes or rice and your choice of vegetable.

* * *

Quick tip 1: Make the food she likes. When your cooking skills improve, you will be able to make everything else look like her favorite foods. Does she like ice cream? Mashed potatoes and pureed peas scooped in a waffle cone anyone? Does she like pie? You can sneak a whole lot of nutritional goodness between the pre-made pie crusts. Worried about fiber, what about sweet potato pie?

Quick tip 2: Put snacks out where she can find them to nibble on. Slightly sweet or lightly salty snacks just before a meal will get her to salivate and prepare her for eating. If you are worried about the salt and sugar, set out carrots, savory mini muffins, graham crackers, cubes of cheese, cut up hot dogs or celery. They must be finger food sized.

Prior to figuring this out, my father ate a bag of cough drops. He thought they were hard candies. Before dinner he showed flu-like symptoms and then lost his dinner. It took a few episodes before we realized what the source was and the cause. I learned to put out snacks. It is okay to let her nibble even if she gains a little weight. Very few people with A.D. are overweight when they pass.

Quick tip 3: If you are having troubles getting her to the dinner table, invite her to join you for dinner. It will make her feel important. Then hand her a warm washcloth to freshen up before the meal. (Wet a washcloth, fold it in half, and roll it up in a tight roll. Put it in the microwave. Depending on the power of your microwave it may only take 30 seconds to warm. Make sure it is not too hot.) If she seems confused, do one for yourself so she can see how to freshen up.

* * *

Color Contrasting the Dishes and Silverware from the Food

One of the issues in later stages of dementia, particularly Alzheimer's Disease (A.D.), is your loved one will eat less and less food. About 40% of people with A.D. lose a significant amount of weight.[68] Because their brain function causes their eyesight to diminish and gives them tunnel vision, they cannot always see what is right in front of them because there is not enough contrast. Dehydration is another issue for people with dementia and has serious health effects.

In the chapter *Preparing Your Living Environment for Your Loved One*, we discussed using contrasting colors to help your loved one maintain their independence and ability to navigate in their surroundings. Researcher Alice Cronin-Golomb, Ph.D. Director, Vision & Cognition Laboratory and Director for Clinical Biopsychology at Boston University, completed two studies on the ability of people with advanced A.D. who were still able to feed themselves. What she found was that using plates, cups, and silverware with a high color contrast to the food on them increased the amount of food and liquid a person with A.D. ate. If the plates, cups, and silverware were red, the participants in the study ate an average of 27 percent more food and drank 83.7 percent more fluids. If the plates, cups, and silverware were blue, they ate an average of 25.1 percent more food and 29.8 percent more liquid.[69]

Cronin-Golomb discovered during the study pastel-colored plates did not have enough contrast to help someone with A.D. to find their food to eat it.

If you want her to finish her food and drink her liquids, dress up the table with solid red or blue-colored plates, cups, and silverware. You can use plastic utensils.

What to Avoid and What to Do:

- Avoid using glassware that may break
- Avoid using dishware with any type of pattern on it
- If she is having confusion over silverware, supply only one utensil, a spoon or spork may work best with an adaptive foam rubber handle for easy gripping. At some point she will only eat with her hands because she can no longer manage the utensil. Do not scold her when she starts doing this, encourage her. It means she can still self-feed and you don't have to feed her yet

- Reduce the number of distractions during mealtime by turning off the television, putting away cell phones, and stop playing video games
- Take her to the bathroom before eating. This will reduce fidgeting and wandering off during the meal
- Does she do better when following the examples of other people at the table or does she eat more when she is by herself?
- Is she confused by the condiments on the table? If yes, remove the salt and pepper, etc.
- Don't put the condiments where she can reach them. Her judgment is impaired, she may pour half a container of salt or sugar on her food
- Once she reaches moderate dementia, the days of the TV tray are over, and she will need to be seated at a table or breakfast counter for stability
- Some people become confused if there are too many food choices on the plate. If that is the case, serve her in courses, in small portions, so she doesn't have to figure out what to eat. For example, meat or fish first, a starchy food like potatoes followed by fruit or vegetables. Let her finish each portion before you put the next one in front of her
- Serve soup in coffee cups or mugs. It is easier to drink the soup from the mug when she can no longer use a spoon
- Cut up all her food into bite sized pieces before you put the plate in front of her. People with late moderate to severe dementia often forget to chew and no longer have the coordination to cut their food on their own. When she gets to this point, make sure the food is soft enough she doesn't have to chew. At some point you will need to puree her food. This will reduce any choking hazards

Now for the meal messiness issue. If dust fears to tread on your floors, you are going to have to find a self-care/respite outlet to vent your frustrations. When mealtime comes, her lost skills may throw your patience out the window, down the block, and into the ravine, where it will land next to the abandoned refrigerator. Plates will get knocked off the table, cups over-filled or knocked over, food will get pushed off plates onto the table or floor as she tries to use a fork or spoon.

There are some things you can do to reduce the messiness:

- Solid color plastic tablecloths or placemats for easy clean-up of spills
- Dycem is a non-slip material that comes in many solid colors. It is washable and reusable. It can hold plates and cups in place, so they don't slide off the table. Dycem is available online, at medical supply houses, or at some large retailers
- Plates with suction cups to hold them in place. These are available online

- Plate guards that attach to the lip of the plates or use scoop plates with suction bases. They reduce the amount of food that slides off the plate and are available online or medical supply stores
- Adding foam rubber to the handle of your silverware, making it larger and easier to manipulate, may extend her using silverware as her coordination declines, especially if she has arthritis

Bibs, Smocks, Aprons

There will be a lot of food spilled down her front. Don't ever use a bib. It implies she is a baby and not an adult. If she is willing to wear either a smock or an apron while dining this will make it easier to get off her and wash regularly. You may need to wear one at the table also, so she won't take if off before eating. For example, if you incorporate the apron into her Sundowners distraction routine, where she sets the table or has a task in the kitchen, getting her to wear it might never be an issue and may help her feel useful. Be sure to thank her for her help. Then let her know she can relax because dinner will be ready in 20 minutes.

If she is on a puréed-food diet because of choking hazards, use a blender or baby food grinder. Puréeing one of the home cooked meals you made from the recipes earlier in this chapter will taste much more appealing than baby food and will save you money in the long run by not purchasing extra food.

Spoon-feeding

If you've never spoon fed anyone, there are a few things to keep in mind. Don't pile the food onto the spoon. Put a small amount of food on the spoon, enough food to fill half the spoon's length. If you put too much on the spoon, she may close her mouth too soon causing some of the food to fall off the spoon. Give her time to chew and swallow before offering her the next bite. At some point you may have to remind her to swallow her food. If she is not eating or is spitting out her food, it could be her mouth or throat are too dry—usually due to medication. Offer her a sip of fluid between each bite to help her swallow her food or mix her food with water or juice.

Check with her pharmacist regarding which medications may cause dry mouth.

Fluid Intake

People with dementia may not remember to drink fluids. Getting them to drink enough fluid, whether it is water or juice is important to prevent issues like dehydration and delirium. Even folks with mild cognitive impairment can forget to drink enough fluids and may need subtle reminders like seeing you sipping on a beverage in front of them. It's called mirroring, if they see you do it, they will usually copy the action.

There are certain fluids they should not have more than one cup of such as caffeinated beverages: coffee, cocoa, colas, hot chocolate, tea. Caffeine is a diuretic, which means it will give her more frequent trips to the bathroom while stealing the precious fluids she needs. Don't give her caffeine in the afternoon as it will worsen the Sundowning behaviors. If you do serve her hot beverages, make sure they are not too hot before you give them to her. She may no longer be able to judge when something is too hot and burn herself.

Anything that will reduce your workload and increase her independence is a win-win.

Swallowing and Pneumonia

With the progression of dementia, swallowing may become an issue. She may carry food around in her mouth because she can't remember to chew or swallow. With the deterioration of her coordination, when she does swallow, she may breathe the food into her lungs instead. It is important to make sure she swallows her food properly.

Breathing food into the lungs is the most common cause of pneumonia in people with dementia. The technical term is aspiration pneumonia. It is the leading cause of death among Alzheimer's patients. The National Institute on Aging (NIH) estimates that the reported cause of death from pneumonia in 2010 was overstated, with 500,000 deaths actually due to Alzheimer's Disease, for which pneumonia was a symptom of the disease, not the actual cause of death.[70]

* * *

Strength is the ability to break a chocolate bar into four pieces with your bare hands and then eat just one of those pieces. –Judith Viorst

Make sure you schedule yourself regular respite time every few days, even if it is only for a couple of hours, so you can breathe . . . and maintain your strength.

Chapter 14: The Deodorant Date: Why You Need Respite

What's Covered in This Chapter
- Why You Need Couples Respite
  - The Deodorant Date
- What Respite Care Might Look Like if You are Single

According to the Alzheimer's Association, there are about 15 million people caring for someone with dementia in the United States, and millions of others around the world. Seeking help and support from others along the way is a necessity.

For example, there may come a time in your life when you find yourself raising your children and/or grandchildren. Then something happens to your parents and you redefine yourself as one of the millions of Americans who've joined the ranks of the Sandwich Generation.

> Sandwich Generation: a generation of people responsible for bringing up their own children or grandchildren and caring for their aging parents.

What if you don't have children? Now you are responsible for "raising" one or both of your parents. Welcome to the Open-Faced Sandwich Generation.

Up to this point, you have no experience but what the school of hard knocks teaches you about managing or administering medication, dealing with finances, legal issues, Medicare, and long-term care insurance—if you're lucky—or even long-term illness beyond aging.

What about the emotional side: maintaining your parents' dignity while maintaining your own sanity? Not to mention the emotional jerk from role reversal and grieving the loss of the relationship to dementia.

Perhaps you're familiar with the axiom, "when you get old, you get cold." Maybe you've never noticed an elderly person walking down the street wearing two sweaters on a seventy-five-degree day. Or if you're like me, you didn't link the two together. Because I didn't make the link, I called the fire department on the first night after my father moved into my home because I didn't recognize the symptoms of hypothermia. We laugh about that one now. At least I now know a hot shower and an electric blanket works wonders.

After you've established the rules of the household for your loved one with dementia, which is another uncomfortable conversation, then there is the transition in your relationships with your significant other. In my case, the relationship with my husband.

Even if your parents or in-laws are congenial, there is still potential for conflict. It is easy to let your relationship with your mate fall apart when you're exhausted from working, caregiving, and maintaining a household.

The goal: Not to take it out on your loved ones and keep your sense of humor.

Why You Need Couples Respite

You've worked a long day, work was chaotic. You're in the kitchen cooking dinner. Your parent, who can no longer help with meal prep, is sitting at the kitchen counter—drumming her fingers—waiting for the meal. You have visions of beating her with a sock puppet named Phil after she's asked you for the third time when will dinner be ready.

It would be too easy to take it out on your unsuspecting mate when they enter the kitchen and ask the same question.

Now is the moment to take a step back, reframe, and realize it doesn't have to be this way. (For more information on the Reframing Technique see the *Distraction Techniques* Chapter page 110.)

> **Reframing** is a technique used in cognitive behavioral therapy to create a different way of looking at a situation, person, or relationship by changing its meaning.

My husband and I work from home, which means we worked, and gave care 24/7.

Enter healthy selfishness. Do you remember the thrill of sneaking out of the house when you were growing up? That adrenaline rush, thinking you might get caught? Maybe you never snuck out.

Sometimes sneaking out of the house after your family member has gone to bed, for twenty or thirty minutes of "quality alone time," lifts the spirits. I'm not advocating abandoning your family member, I am suggesting taking twenty or thirty minutes of respite to keep your relationship with your mate alive and healthy.

The Deodorant Date

We called these "deodorant dates" because that's what we needed at the store the first time we took one. We chased each other around the store—slowly so we would not get caught. Only we got caught. Yeah, we live in a small town, so from that point on when the staff of our local grocer saw the two of us in the store without my father chaperoning, a member of the staff would ask us if this was our "deodorant date."

A few moments of shared romance can lift pounds of stress off your shoulders. It could be as simple as running down the street holding hands, laughing, and looking over your shoulders to see if anyone saw you. Or having a family member or friend spend some time with your loved one while you go to the local drive-in burger joint, have a burger, and neck in the back seat of the car. Do whatever works for your relationship.

If Tom Sawyer can convince his friends that whitewashing a fence is fun, you should be able to convince your mate that a date is what you make it. Even if it's just a quick run to the grocery store for deodorant.

What Respite Care Might Look Like if You are Single

By focusing so much on your loved one's needs, it is so easy to stop taking care of your own health. When you stop taking care of yourself, it hurts you and the person you are caring for if you do not get enough down time. It is important to ask for help. Reach out to other family members, friends, church members, or volunteer organizations for help with the day-to-day caregiving. The help could be something like cleaning, grocery shopping, or someone who is chatty "visiting" for an hour or two with your loved one. It could even include adult day care services or forming a caregiving group like *Share the Care* (see *Knowing Your Own Limitations Before You Make the Decision for Care*, page 15).

If someone is there spending time with your loved one, you will have time for well-earned rest and relaxation. Maybe take in a movie with a friend, sit in a park and read a book or just people watch, or run an errand by yourself. Run through a sprinkler, blow bubbles, go for a walk or to the gym, or work on an art or craft project. Be sure to include something that keeps your creativity and spirit alive. If family members or friends are willing to stay with your loved one for a few days, take a road trip.

Dementia care is very isolating. You may feel you are being disloyal to your loved one if someone else spends some time with her. That is not the case, your loved one needs to be social as much as you do. It is too easy to get into the mindset that you have to do it all or it won't get done right. Asking for help is not a sign of weakness. When someone offers help, accept it. Accept that you have value and you deserve the down time. Caregivers who take respite provide better care and find more satisfaction in caregiving. Now go have some fun.

Chapter 15: Elder Abuse

According to AARP, 1 in 10 Americans aged 60 and over have experienced some form of elder abuse. But even as prosecutors around the country target elder abuse, many cases go unreported. Some older adults fear that if they complain, they will end up in a nursing home.

According to the National Adult Protective Services Association, it is estimated that only 1 in 44 cases of senior financial abuse are ever reported.

What is Elder Abuse?

Elder abuse is generally defined as the mistreatment of older persons in home or institutional settings. At the time of this writing there is no uniform definition. In general, it is defined as any unnecessary suffering, whether it is self-inflicted or inflicted by others, that negatively affects an older person's quality of life.

The four most common types of elder abuses are neglect, financial/material abuse, psychological/emotional abuse and physical abuse that includes sexual abuse.[71]

Neglect comes in a couple of forms: passive or active. Active neglect is the intentional deprivation of goods or services necessary to maintain a person's physical or mental health. Passive neglect is the failure to recognize an older person's needs, which results in keeping them from getting the goods or services they require.

Financial and material abuse includes any behavior by a relative or caregiver, without the knowledge or consent of the older person. This results in financial exploitation through illegal or unethical use of their money or property or other assets for the relative or caregiver's personal gain.

Psychological and emotional abuse includes threats or acts directed at an older person which invoke fear of violence or isolation that may result in depression, mental anguish, or anxiety.

Physical abuse includes bodily harm of an elderly person, injury, unnecessary pain, mental distress, unreasonable confinement, coercion, or punishment. Sometimes signs of physical abuse are not obvious and might be camouflaged with clothing or blankets.

Sexual abuse includes any form of unwanted sexual contact that results from threats, force, or inability of the older person to give their consent. This includes assault, rape, and sexual harassment.

It's important to remember that violence and the related behaviors are learned and passed down from one generation to the next. It is not uncommon for a child who was abused by their parent to become abusive as an adult. Then as the caregiver for their parents, they may take it out on the aging parent and even extend it to their own spouse or children.

Victims of elder abuse frequently present symptoms similar to victims of battered child or battered wife syndrome.

Some of the things to watch for are unexplained injuries or repeated injuries such as cuts, burns, and broken or dislocated bones, unexplained rapid weight-loss, withdrawal from social situations not caused by dementia, evidence their medical needs are not being met such as bedsores or lack of personal cleanliness, monies missing from bank accounts or missing assets, and fear of certain family members or caregivers.

Many times, abuse occurs because the family member chosen to provide care is the least capable of doing the caregiving. Compound that with your loved one not being able to remember they have been abused. Those who would be their advocate, other family members, often live hundreds or even thousands of miles away, and are not there to help them.

For example, Jessie, whose name has been changed to protect her family members' privacy, shared her experience with financial elder abuse.

> *Henry was the golden-haired youngest grandchild, and clearly my mother-in-law's favorite. He charged items to his grandmother's credit card online. The charges weren't large amounts, and my brother-in-law told him to stop. My in-laws were not worried. In fact, my mother-in-law refused to hear a single critical word about him and dismissed her adult children's concerns.*
>
> *When Henry couldn't live with family friends, grandparents or either divorced parent, Child Protective Services was called in. Henry lived with us for nine months. It was marked by lying, cheating in school, dragging friends into the situation, binge drinking, secretly opening bank accounts, and frequent demands for high-end items. He moved back to the Midwest at the school's year end, to our relief.*
>
> *The entire family was surprised to hear he'd be attending a state university in Arizona, about 150 miles from where my husband's parents wintered every year. We thought he'd been awarded a scholarship based on need. All of us hoped for the best.*
>
> *Not long after, my mother-in-law passed away from a stroke. My husband and I travelled to Arizona to help his father, who struggled with the early signs of Alzheimer's disease. We learned Henry visited with several of his fraternity friends, drinking and carousing, while his grandfather sat at his wife's bedside as her body shut down.*

Before the memorial service, we cleaned up paperwork scattered throughout the house. We discovered documents from the university's office of financial aid — our nephew was no longer a student.

Henry was admitted to the university by applying for financial aid and forging his grandfather's name and signature, using his grandfather's Social Security number and other personal financial information. Later, he told his grandfather he "needed money right away or the university wouldn't let him into college." My father-in-law authorized payments through his financial planner.

Our nephew defrauded the U.S. Department of Education of funds he never used for education and stole over $80,000 from his grandfather.

We notified credit card companies and credit reporting agencies along with law enforcement authorities in several states. It was not deemed a high priority crime and not pursued. What hurt our family most was his betrayal of trust and lack of remorse.

There are many things that you can do in a situation like this to reduce or prevent the abuse. Here's what to look for and what you can do.

Warning Signs of Financial Fraud for Vulnerable Seniors:

- Look for unpaid bills or letters and calls from collection agencies
- Bank statements may stop arriving because they are being diverted to another address
- Personal property goes missing
- Signatures on checks and legal documents look suspicious
- Correspondence related to new bank accounts being set up
- A large numbers of credit card offers arrive in the mail or by email
- Strange or implausible explanations are provided by the senior or their caregiver concerning financial transactions and assets

What You Can do to Protect Your Loved Ones

- Appoint a responsible family member to monitor the vulnerable senior's accounts or hire an independent third party such as a member of the American Association of Daily Money Managers to monitor bank accounts and credit cards. Their website is http://secure.aadmm.com. A certified financial planner may also have helpful resources
- Hold regular family meetings with the adult children to make sure everyone's on the same page about how finances are being handled and who has authority to issue checks and transfer funds

- Alert the senior's bank manager at their local branch to be on the lookout for unusual activity. You may need a financial power of attorney to do this, depending on the laws in your state
- Sign your loved one up for a credit monitoring service
- Register your loved one's telephone number on the National Do Not Call Registry. This won't prevent phone scams, but it will reduce the number of calls requesting donations
- Set up a United States Postal Service Informed Delivery account for your loved one to monitor the incoming mail, website: https://informeddelivery.usps.com/box/pages/intro/start.action. This free service allows you to see what is arriving in the mail each day to monitor for fraudulent activities
- Set up a durable financial power of attorney for your loved one or yourself if there are concerns about the ability to manage financial affairs

A durable financial power of attorney allows someone of your loved one's choosing to manage their finances in the event they are unable to make the decisions for themselves, due to something like an illness or dementia. The official title of the person named varies by state, but they are often referred to as an agent or attorney-in-fact.

Your loved one sets the limits on what their agent can do for them. When deciding what an agent can do for them, they may need some of the following taken care of if they are out of commission:

- Paying bills
- Paying taxes
- Paying medical bills*
- Managing any real estate
- Revising their will
- Accessing their bank accounts
- Managing their investments
- Collecting their retirement benefits
- Selling or transferring their assets to pay bills
- Purchasing needed insurance
- Managing or selling their small business
- Hiring someone to represent them, such as an attorney

*If the person they appoint as durable financial power of attorney is not the same person as their durable medical power of attorney, there is a potential for conflict. If the agents disagree over medical care, the financial agent can make getting medical care very difficult.

There is a distinction between durable and regular power of attorney, whether financial power of attorney or regular power of attorney. Power of attorney only allows the person to carry out the loved one's wishes while they are still capable. Once the loved one is incapacitated, they will not have the power to carry out their wishes. Durable powers of attorney remain in effect when your loved one is incapacitated. Other ways it can be made invalid are through divorce, if the person named is not available or unwilling to participate, if a court invalidates it, or your loved one chooses to revoke it.

If you are caring for a spouse with dementia and choose to divorce during the course of dementia for financial reasons, you will no longer have any authority to make decisions for her. Consult an attorney before making the decision.

Most states have forms you can fill out to make someone a financial agent. While most states don't require the use of their forms, their forms will offer the most protection under state law. The forms will need to be signed, witnessed, and notarized. The witness cannot be the person you are naming as an agent.

If you have any questions about power of attorney, get legal help.

As with all powers of attorney, they end automatically at the time of passing.

How to Report Financial Elder Abuse

Reporting financial elder abuse varies from state to state. In most cases, your local law enforcement agency has forms you can fill out to report your concerns. When you are making a report, either written or verbal, you will need to supply the following information to law enforcement:

- The name of the elder being abused
- Their home address, which includes long term care facilities
- The name of the suspected abuser
- The suspected abuser's home address
- The location(s) where the suspected event took place. This will determine who investigates. If it happens in a nursing home, adult family home, or assisted living facility then the Long-Term Care Ombudsman Program would handle the report. If it happens in a private home, then Adult Protective Services (APS) would investigate
- Give specific details about the suspected event, include what you saw or heard that made you suspect fraud. Make copies of all relevant documents, if possible. Using the example above you could say "My nephew, Henry Smith, used his grandfather's Social Security number and other personal financial information to

gain access to his bank accounts. I heard him threaten his grandmother so he could purchase a MacBook."

You are not required to give your name or contact information. If you are afraid of the suspected abuser, you may be able to stay anonymous. Providing your name may help those investigating your claim. Law enforcement needs witnesses in order to build a case against an abuser. If you know of any other witnesses of the suspected abuse, share their names with law enforcement.

How to Report Physical Elder Abuse

People who witness elder abuse should call 9-1-1. There is a state-by-state list of where to report elder abuse at the U.S. Administration on Aging's National Center. The National Center on Elder Abuse website: https://ncea.acl.gov/Resources/State.aspx.

Additional help may be found at the following:

National Adult Protective Services Association:
http://www.napsa-now.org/get-help/help-in-your-area/

National Council on Child Abuse & Family Violence:
https://www.preventfamilyviolence.org/adult-protective-services-numbers

National Long-Term Care Ombudsman Resource Center:
http://theconsumervoice.org/get_help
This website is for use with nursing home, assisted living facilities, or adult family homes.

If you need an attorney who is certified in elder law, the following websites have databases of attorneys listed by state:

The National Elder Law Foundation lists attorneys who are certified in elder law by state. Website: https://nelf.org/search/custom.asp?id=5427

The National Academy of Elder Law Attorneys website: http://www.naela.org/.

Ways to Avoid Elder Abuse

Caregiver burnout can lead to abuse. Feeling unprepared for caregiving responsibilities, the uncertainties of how to be help someone with dementia, and the financial stresses all play a part.[72] There are ways to reduce the stress.

- Spot your own emotional triggers, for example impatience or feeling out of control. Once you recognize your triggers, you will know when to give yourself a time-out before you do something you might regret

- Counseling. It's a great way to vent your emotional spleen and teaches you how to manage emotional triggers

- Join a support group. If you don't know where to search, see *Knowing When to Say When* on page 166, or look at the *Resources* section at the end of this book, see page 221

- Find community resources. See the *Resources* section for a list of websites, page 215

- Share the caregiving burden. The more people you involve in caregiving the less stress you will create for yourself. Ask family members, friend, neighbors, or co-workers. You never know where help will come from unless you ask. You might even receive help you didn't even expect. See *Knowing Your Own Limitations Before You Make the Decision for Care* for details on the Share the Caregiving program page 15 or visit their website at www.sharethecare.org

- Make time for your personal life. You need time for self-care, hobbies, and social activities. You cannot be "on" 24/7, it's okay to be human. You need hugs, too

Chapter 16:
Reinventing Your Relationship

"One doesn't recognize the really important moments in one's life until it's too late."
~Agatha Christie

Altered Reality and Second Chances

There are many downsides to dementia care, but there are some upsides, too. We all crave connections with our loved ones, and dementia robs us of that connection. Some may never have had a deep connection because their loved one didn't know how to meet that need. Once your loved one reaches the middle to late moderate stage of dementia, her dementia will move her into an earlier portion of her life. She may no longer recognize you, whether you are her spouse, sibling, parent, or child. She may think you are someone else, like her sister, brother, aunt, uncle, friend, or neighbor.

If your lifelong relationship with your loved one was rocky, argumentative, or tenuous, you have an opportunity to reinvent that part of the relationship you longed for because the rules have changed. Their reality changed, their truth changed, and you can choose to meet them in their reality, where they live on their terms, and regain some of the connection you missed out on.

In the chapter *Memory Aids and the Family*, we discussed how to answer questions about family members who have passed away. When she asks you questions like, "Where are my children?" Instead of telling her you are standing right in front of her, figure out where she is in her reality so you can answer her question based on where she is. Use photographs from her life, or ask her who the president is, and she will guide you to the approximate year she is living through. Then you can answer the question by saying:

- "Alex and Andrea are in school."
- "Your baby is napping."
- "Alex is at baseball practice."
- "Andrea is at a sleep-over at the McCloud's tonight."

If she becomes upset by the answer or doesn't believe you, wait a bit until she calms down, then change your answer. Repeat this process until she is happy with the answer. For example, if she thinks her kids are older, perhaps in their twenties, telling her Alex is at baseball practice may not fly unless he is a professional baseball player. But if Alex was working his way through college and she was expecting him to come home for the weekend, you can say something like, "He's at school and will be home this weekend."

If she is looking for a former spouse who cheated on her, she might not accept an answer that Joe is at work, but she might accept he's having a drink at the bar with co-workers . . . and then she might tell you what a louse he is and why she should divorce him. You may hear family stories and revelations you've never heard before, too.

Once you've found the answers that work, write down the answers and tell anyone who visits so they may have a better visit, too.

If she becomes agitated with you and will not calm down, try these steps:

- Leave the room
- Change your clothes, put on a hat, a wig, or put your hair up, and come back into the room as a different person, either dressed as an adult or child
- Gentlemen, if you are taking care of your wife, put on coveralls and look like a plumber, handyman, or dress like a cable repairman. You will be less threatening as the repairman. Make sure you tell her you are the repairman and what you are there for, like repairing the dishwasher. Then you can also offer her any additional help she may need
- Be calm, using a straight-forward approach and get down on her eye level and maintain eye contact, much like you would with a child
- Touch her arm or knee to get her attention
- Introduce yourself using your first name. If this causes her an issue, perhaps use your middle name or a nickname
- Smile and relax
- Speak to her using her first name
- Pay attention to her tone of voice and body language. Watch for more agitation or anxiety
- When speaking about anyone else, do not use the pronouns 'he' or 'she.' They will cause confusion. Always use first names
- Affirm everything she says to you, even if you don't understand what she's saying, with things like, "Tell me more," "You don't say," "Go on," or "Wow, really." Smile and laugh. She may not have a clue what you are saying, but she will respond to your body language and calmness
- Stick to short sentences
- Avoid asking questions unless they are yes or no questions that you can demonstrate with an action. Otherwise she may become confused. For example, "Sarah, I'm going to have a glass of water, would you like to join me?"

- Show a photo of yourself during the time frame she believes she is living in. To start the conversation, let's say you showed her a photo of you riding a bicycle at the age of ten, then say something like, "Sheila sure can ride a bicycle." The beauty of this is it does not require any short-term memory on her part. You may hear some things you've never heard about yourself before such as how proud she is of you, or you may hear things you never wanted to know
- Talk about everything in the present tense. For example, if she was a talented quilter, say "You are a great quilter." Perhaps she loved sailing, hiking, or riding horseback. Even though she can't do it anymore, remind her of her skills in the present tense. For men, perhaps they loved hunting, auto repair, creating realistic costumes and weapons for renaissance fairs, or perhaps even building tree houses, so remind them of what they loved. You may be surprised with a recovered memory
- When you are finished talking, give her a smile or a hug or pat on the back
- If the meltdown continues, walk away and try again later

Take advantage of the do overs dementia gives you for mending your relationship. Give yourself permission to put emotional distance between the two of you. This may be the most difficult thing you will ever try. Not everyone will be able to do this and that is okay. Speak to her like a friend instead of a spouse, sibling, parent, or child, and put the baggage in the basement for a little while to collect some dust. Find a common connection, whether it's watching television game shows, or playing cards, or some other interest. You may get a relationship much deeper than you expected, in ways you never anticipated.

During the last year of my mother's life, she said to me, "They keep telling me you are my daughter, but I don't remember you. I only know you as the Book Lady."

I said, "I am the Book Lady."

In the last year of her life I read to her for a couple of hours every day from Lillian Jackson Braun's "The Cat Who" series. We were able to discuss our shared love of the stories. At the very end when she could no longer speak, I knew I could still connect with her through reading those stories. She passed two days after we finished the series. We made it to "The End."

There are no big victories in caring for someone with dementia. It is the collection of small moments you will remember and cherish. I still laugh when I think of my father when he said, "I've got big hands," holding his hands a few inches from a saleswoman's face while he tried to explain he wanted to buy a pair of gloves. Ten years from now you may remember and laugh about your version of "I've got big hands." You won't know what you are missing unless you try.

Your heart is worth mending. Don't wait until it's too late.

Chapter 17: Knowing When to Say When

"Caregiving sometimes feels like a set of fingernails on the blackboard of life." ~Lou Cook

This life-lesson in caregiving is not meant to crush us but meant to remind us to take care of ourselves, forgive ourselves, accept ourselves, and survive ourselves. Many people battle up this same hill every day wondering: "Is this an old age thing, or does she really need my help?, Am I doing the right thing?, How do I know I am making the best choice?, What is the next step?"

Most of us are thrust into caregiving because we don't recognize there is an issue, we are in denial, or we live too far away to see what is happening. It might be that your loved one is so good at covering up, everything seems fine until it isn't.

My journey started when my father couldn't handle being my mother's caregiver anymore. At that time, there was an in-home aid assisting him for four hours, five days a week, so he could get time to himself to run errands and get some down time. It wasn't enough.

He reached burnout, and we didn't recognize the signs or even know what to watch for or how to check in on him. He was irritable and snappish. His anger simmered below the surface. He would fall asleep the moment he sat in a chair and snacked on candy to get him through the day. Because he stopped taking care of his diabetes, he lived on aspirin to cover the headaches from the excess sugar. He looked for any chance to get away from home. When asked how he was doing, he always said, "I am fine." I discovered too late "fine" did not describe his emotional or physical state. It was a pat answer to side-step the question. He felt he should be stronger than he was and waited too long to ask for help.

Covering up is a normal part of caregiving and a normal part of dementia.

In caregiving, it is when the caregiver does not want to express their negative feelings for fear they will be judged by others or themselves, or don't want to burden others with their problems.[73]

In dementia, especially Alzheimer's Disease, the affected person is covering up what they are forgetting, pretending that all is normal, because they want to be seen as normal.

When the time came, I quit my job so I could take care of my mom. In less than two weeks my family and I were making decisions we never considered before, including long-term care, and end-of-life planning. We placed my mother in a care facility.

My mother was asked to leave the first facility at the end of the first month because she required more care than they were staffed to handle. During her one month stay, she declined rapidly and developed three bed sores that exposed her tail bone and spine. Fortunately, the hospice nurse assigned to her care spotted the bed sores and guided us to a facility better suited to my mother's needs. That facility cared for her so well, two of the three sores healed before she died some months later.

There are many different situations that let you know it's time to say when. It could be women who are caring for men and can no longer physically help lift him out of bed, or if the situation becomes abusive, these are indication that it's time to look for outside care. Historically, most men were not typically caregivers, however, more men are taking care of their spouses, mothers, siblings, or partners. When men are caring for women, incontinence is usually when men reach for outside help or placement in a skilled care facility. Incontinence is something men believe they can fix, but they cannot fix it, and it usually causes them to wave the white flag.

Adult children tend to wait the longest to step in, waiting to get permission from their parents that may never come. Perhaps their parents may not want to ask for help, or the adult children don't want to take on the role reversal.

There is no perfect answer for caregiving. The better answer is the one you make, at the time you are making it, with the best information available to you at the time. You can expect any major decision will be difficult, gut wrenching, and wrapped in guilt with a big red bow.

Ask yourself, "How am I doing?" If you're truthful, you will not use the pat answer "I'm fine." That's the one-way ticket down the river "denial," and the fastest road to burnout. Preferably family members and friends will check in with you regularly to make sure you haven't crossed the burnout bridge.

For example, Gina, whose name has been changed to protect her family's privacy, shared her experience with denial.

> I think I was in denial for a long time with my mom. She probably should've gone into a care facility sooner than she did. She had always been such a take-charge type. It was hard for me to realize that she couldn't do that anymore. But I guess when I really realized we had to do something was when I'd go over and sort all her pills for the week into a pill box for each day, and the next day they would all be mushed up in one or two of the little boxes and full of water.
>
> She was really good at covering for herself, and since I was in denial, we made a bad team. One day my aunt went to see her. My mom was having some sort of mental

episode. She hunkered under the dining room table, afraid for her life. Someone was coming in to kill her. She came out of it once she heard my aunt's voice. That's when I realized she needed more care.

She was living in a senior apartment. We moved her to a care facility. That facility said they'd take care of her meds and keep an eye on her. They didn't do what they were supposed to, and she went downhill. Not that she wouldn't have anyway, but they didn't help. They fought with her instead of helping her. About three months before she died, we moved her into memory care. That decision was taken out of my hands because the other place told me I had to move her. She was not pleased. When she "came to" and realized she was locked in, she was mad at me. I think at that point she just gave up.

It was such a tough time for me. Being the youngest, and the only girl, everything was left for me to do. All the decisions, all the care, and I was the one who took her out for visits and shopping, etc. I had to plan her funeral alone. I still haven't forgiven my brothers for that. My brothers were pretty worthless, except they did support my decisions, so I guess I should be thankful for that.

Once you suspect you are out of your depth, it's time to look into alternative care for your loved one. For example, in-home health care by an aide or skilled nurse, group care like Share the Care (see *Knowing Your Own Limitations Before You Make the Decision for Care* page 15) or Village to Village Network (see *Resources* page 218). Village to Village Network is an organization who helps communities start Villages. Villages are membership-based groups who respond to the needs of older people within a geographic area.   Other examples for care are the relocation of your loved one to assisted living, a memory care facility, or a skilled nursing facility.

Knowing when to say when and when to ask for help is *not failure*. Failure is not asking for help and the harm that befalls one or both of you, including injury, illness, or death.

The Signs of Caregiver Burnout

None of us have superhuman abilities. We are human, have specific talents, and have limits to our strength and resources. Caregiving for someone with dementia isn't easy. You need to know what burnout looks like.[74] If you notice any of the following signs, reach out for help:

- Trouble falling asleep or staying asleep each night for more than two weeks
- Frequent nightmares
- Irritability
- Impatience
- Mood swings

- Feeling anxious
- Feeling resentment
- High levels of stress
- Difficulty concentrating
- Exhaustion
- Inability to cope with one or more problems and feeling overwhelmed
- Increased need for sugar
- Significant weight loss or weight gain
- Digestive issues
- Blowing up over minor incidents like a spilled glass of water or children playing
- Back aches, body pains, or headaches that make you rely on over-the-counter pain relievers or prescription drugs
- Other health problems that have you trying to remember when the last time was you felt good
- Medicating with recreational drugs or alcohol
- Start smoking, start smoking again after quitting, or smoking more than previously. This includes vaping
- Losing interest in normal activities
- Losing hope
- A feeling of failure
- Feeling isolated
- Thoughts of running away
- Cannot laugh or feel joy
- Frequently crying or feeling sad
- Loss of compassion
- Feeling trapped
- Thinking of suicide

You may have made the time in your schedule for respite, but there may come a time when you can no longer manage the caregiving without additional help. You may also feel guilty because your loved one made you promise never to put her in a nursing home or never to let her get "that way." In many cases, that is the impossible promise.

Asking for help will help you survive caregiving.

Stages of Care

There are three stages of dementia care. Each stage contains its own challenges.

Mild Cognitive Decline

This is the time to begin defining your limits. Only you know what you can and cannot handle. Before you are feeling angry, lost, out of control, or showing signs of burnout, consider the following:

Support Groups

They come in all shapes and sizes. They don't make you talk if you aren't comfortable doing so. It's best to test them out first to see if you fit in. If you are hearing lots of "aha's" among the group members and you feel the same way in that moment, this might be the group for you. If you don't have that feeling, or you have progressed beyond the level of the support group, try another.

Not everyone can make it to support groups. If you have internet access, there are support groups available online.

Support groups aren't for everyone. For those more comfortable in an informational seminar or session, local hospitals often offer these services as well as local Alzheimer's Association chapters.

Try checking with your local Alzheimer's Association for local groups at https://alz.org/help-support/community/support-groups or for the online forum, go to https://www.alzconnected.org/.

Grief Counselling for Dementia Care

Do you know what grief looks like for you? It will be different for everyone. Before your eyes, you are losing someone you depended upon for emotional support, connection, and even validation. Someone who helped you get through difficult times, shared projects with you, and laughed with you. It doesn't happen all at once. It happens slowly. First you find yourself getting annoyed at the little things. Then you catch them in "a lie," or poor decisions and you become angry. Only the lie isn't a lie, it's their dementia altering their reality.

Let's say you snap after one too many "lies," or poor decisions and you refuse to help them unless they ask for help. This might be what your grief looks like.

Grief counselling may help you recognize it's the disease and not your loved one. It may help you regain your compassion and perspective and ease the burden of long-term loss.

The Psychology Today website contains a detailed list of mental health professionals in the United States by state. Their website is: https://www.psychologytoday.com/us/therapists/grief. Check with your health insurance or, if eligible, with Medicare to find out what is covered for you. Some programs have online counseling or telephone-based counseling which may be helpful and more affordable.

For more information on managing grief and guilt, see the blog post: *Grief and Loss and Guilt with Dementia* on my website tracycramperkins.com/blog.

Health and Home Aides

Help comes in many forms. The following list may give you ideas of where to turn for help and the search terms to use when you search the web:

- **Adult Day Care for Dementia**: it offers both medical and social services including activities for your loved one
- **Chore Services**: these services run errands, make household repairs, and do yardwork
- **Group Meals**: these services, usually run by local churches, senior centers, or other charitable organizations, offer a nutritious meal and a chance to socialize
- **Home-delivery Meals**: these are prepared meals delivered to those who can no longer cook or shop for themselves. Check with local Senior Centers or your local Area Agency on Aging to locate the services available in your area
- **Home Health Aide Services**: these services offer assistance with medications, exercise, and personal care, such as bathing
- **Occupational Therapy**: occupational therapists treat people to improve their functional abilities, such as cooking, cleaning, and mobility
- **Paid Companion**: this is someone who comes to your home and provides supervision, personal care, and socializing when the primary caregiver is not there
- **Telephone Support**: you, a family member, or trusted friend make regular phone calls to the person who is isolated or homebound
- **Transportation**: transportation services for getting to medical appointments and elsewhere.

Moderate Cognitive Decline

The signs of burnout will become more obvious at this stage of care. You may feel angry, depressed, or hopeless. You may be sleep deprived. Your need for self-care and respite are a necessity. Pay attention to your body's signs of stress, including your blood pressure.

By this time, you may have forgotten what it means to take care of yourself, such as eating regular nutritious meals, getting sleep, and regular exercise. Consider adding twenty minutes of Yoga, Tai chi, Qigong, meditation, or perhaps even a trip to the spa for a massage once a week.

There are breathing exercises to help you reduce your stress. Set aside several times a day to ground yourself with breathing exercise. Set a timer on your smart phone to remind yourself to take five-minute time-outs to breathe. Learn to accept your emotions, good or bad, instead of wishing they didn't exist. A good support group can really help.

Now is the time when family, friends, neighbors, or people from church can help by visiting with your loved one or cooking a meal or cleaning so you can take care of yourself. One of the best gifts you can give them is teaching them how to visit so you can get some respite. If you haven't created a routine list for your loved one yet, do what one of my friends did with the following letter to help their friends and family. Their names have been changed to protect their privacy.

Dear family and friends,

As you know, Elaine has Alzheimer's and it is getting tougher for us to come see you. We enjoy your friendship and wanted to share some tips for visiting us.

Elaine has some good days and some tough days. If possible, would you please call me ahead of time so I can let you know what kind of day it is? If it's a tough day, the visit may be very short or not at all. On a good day, stay and enjoy yourself for a while. I may excuse myself from the party to get some time to myself.

I know you would like to visit as a family but more than two people visiting overwhelms Elaine as does too much noise or lots of conversation at the same time. If you are loud, don't be surprised if she loses it and yells at you. It's the Alzheimer's talking.

When you see her, greet her with a hug and a smile. If you want to bring her a treat, she is still addicted to olives and cherries, but can't have any with pits. She still likes ice cream sandwiches and looking at photo albums and scrapbooks. If you have any pictures with Elaine and family or friends, sharing them with her may give her a memory back for a short time.

She still enjoys crafting but now the projects are very simple. If you want to do a project with her, she would be very happy. She also enjoys going for car rides, listening to swing and jazz, or being read to from her favorite books. Sometimes she likes to sit quietly. If that's the case, hold her hand, it will mean the world to her.

If you take her out to eat without me, avoid overly crowded restaurants or the lunch rush. I can also suggest "safe" restaurants. She can't order for herself anymore, so before you leave, I will give you a list of what she likes to order.

She wants to be part of the conversation and can still participate. She may repeat a story several times, so please be patient. She sometimes has trouble with words. If you don't understand what she is saying, just agree with her and smile or wink or both.

Please don't ask any questions that make her use her short-term memory, like "Do you remember . . . ?" Instead tell her about the things you have been doing. If she gets frustrated, order dessert. If you're at our house, I keep the freezer stocked with ice cream sandwiches. Her mood is always lifted with a sweet treat, but limit the coffee to one cup of leaded, or two cups unleaded. I will thank you for it later.

Thank you for accepting us in this new life we find ourselves in. Each day is different, and we hope you will join us.

With our thanks and love,

Jim and Elaine†

You can write your letter like this one, covering your loved one's needs, and share it with family and friends.

†According to Jim, his letter was modeled after an example from Jolene Brackey's book, *Creating Moments of Joy Along the Alzheimer's Journey.*

* * *

Severe Cognitive Decline

What are the End-of-Life Care Goals?

No two dementia care experiences are the same. The older a person is when they get dementia means they are more likely to pass away from another condition like cancer or heart disease rather than from dementia. Sometimes when your loved one goes from moderate to severe Alzheimer's Disease they may die quickly if they fall and break a hip. This is because being bedridden seems to cause further decline in their dementia and possibly pneumonia, or they have a stroke which causes paralysis. The final downturn can be rapid. Or they decline, rally and repeat until they slowly dwindle away. This is known as the dwindles. Someone with early onset dementia will usually pass from the disease itself. Those with early onset may also experience the dwindles.

> *The dwindles* are a condition of physical deterioration involving several body systems shutting down.

This stage of care becomes an emotional roller coaster, second guessing yourself, not sleeping, and constant worry, in addition to juggling work and family life. Trying to balance your loved one's wishes with your own emotional needs, and not having the skill set to handle the additional burden of care can be exhausting for any family member.

Your loved one's doctor may now suggest you scale back on the level of care. Certain procedures and treatments are for people who might expect to live another ten years. Those treatments may not be helpful to someone in this stage of dementia. Screenings such as mammograms and colonoscopies at this stage of dementia would do more harm than help.[75] When someone is frail, certain forms of treatment may even be harmful, for example, cardiopulmonary resuscitation (CPR) may break ribs. Someone with dementia can suffer from the side effects of some medications—especially general anesthetics, which may cause her condition to worsen, as can the trauma of emergency care.

This will be the most emotionally wrenching part of your caregiving journey. If your loved one did not make her advanced wishes known, you will be making several end-of-life care decisions. However, certain medical interventions will offer fewer benefits, meaning they won't extend the quality or quantity of her life. So it makes sense to scale back care.

Most people with dementia do not die at home. In the last few months, hospitalization becomes more frequent or they may end up in a skilled nursing facility recovering from a fall or a stroke.

Before a medical crisis occurs at this stage of dementia, think about what your goals are for her care. Do you want to extend her life, give her the ability to function better, or improve her level of comfort? With the worsening of Alzheimer's disease, doing all three will not be possible. Which aspect will you choose? Did she already express her wishes in her durable power of medical attorney document or when filling out a P.O.L.S.T. with her physician? If yes, follow her wishes.

If additional treatments are suggested, ask her doctor the following questions prior to deciding:[76]

- What happens if we wait and watch the condition?
- What will happen if we do not treat it?
- Is there an easier treatment? If yes, what are the side effects of going with the treatment?
- How stressful is the test procedure?
- How stressful is the treatment?

Before deciding, ask your doctor how long she is expected to live. Keep in mind some doctors may not want to tell you everything that is going on with her because it will be hard for you to hear and it is a hard question to ask. The benefit of asking the question is it may prevent unnecessary or uncomfortable treatments.

Things to consider when deciding when and how you might scale back care:[77]

- Should your loved one be screened for cancer? Will she be able to handle the procedure? If the procedure requires an MRI, PET Scan, CAT Scan, x-rays, or other similar screening, would she be able to hold still that long, or would she fight it?
- When should you stop providing preventative health care? For example, dental visits, eye exams, or medications such as statins

- Should certain symptoms be followed up? If it is an invasive procedure such as treatment for a disease that requires taking samples of breast tissue or spots on the lungs, then no. If it is, for example, a blood draw to determine if there is an infection that could be treated to ease suffering, then it should be done. Always consult your loved one's physician

- When do you reduce trips to or stop going to the hospital? At some point in this stage, hospitalization is not likely to make her feel better but will make her feel worse. Hospitalization and/or intensive care at this stage can trigger the following issues for someone with advanced dementia:
   o Weakness and decline caused by confusion, pain, stress, poor sleep, inactivity and poor nutrition
   o Anxiety
   o Depression

- When do you stop treatments that might help, but are too hard on her? For example, dehydration becomes an issue at this point. For some using an IV for fluids might work well. She might not mind being held in place for an IV, especially if a cannula sleeve is used. For others, it might be too distressing because they can't remember why it is happening and may struggle to free themselves. It may be easier to hydrate by hand with ice chips or water from a dropper

> A **Cannula sleeve** is a knitted sleeve similar to a fidget quilt, which when placed over the arm and the IV needle, allows someone with dementia to fidget with the items attached to the sleeve and leave the IV (Intravenous cannulation—the needle) in their arm.

- When do you stop providing the minimal treatment that no longer provides comfort? You should always take care of pain and constipation. But at this stage of life, treating a urinary tract infection (UTI) may not even provide any comfort. Dementia medications like Aricept, Exelon, Razadyne, or Namenda will not help any longer

Pain

Pain is under-recognized and not often treated in people with dementia. Pain can be caused by a different chronic disease like nerve damage or cancer, from being bedridden and developing bed sores or from the dying process itself. Your loved one may also be going through emotional pain, including feeling anxious about passing.

Unfortunately, those with dementia at this stage don't have the ability to tell you how they are feeling. They may no longer recognize a pain scale, even the ones with faces for words. What you should watch for in those with Alzheimer's Disease:[78]

- Using expressions like, "I don't know," or "Help me," or "It's not right," or "It feels tight."
- Rubbing a body part
- Favoring a body part
- Handwringing
- Rapid blinking
- Moaning
- Crying
- Lashing out
- Agitation
- Other signs of distress or changes in behavior

Palliative Care and Hospice

Misconceptions about Hospice

In an interview with Amanda Reed, BSN, Area Vice President of Business Development, Kindred Hospice, we discussed the common misconceptions surrounding hospice, what people should be aware of when looking for a hospice program, veterans' programs, volunteering, and bereavement support.

Tracy: "What are the top things most people don't know or understand about hospice?"

Amanda: "There are so many misunderstandings about hospice. Here are a few I frequently encounter. Hospice is only for individuals that are very close to dying. This is a myth; hospice is covered for at least 6 months and is 100% paid for by Medicare and private insurances.

Many believe hospice is a place, and many believe that if they begin hospice they have to go to a "hospice house." This, too, is a myth, as hospice is a service that cares for individuals for wherever they call home.

Another common misconception is that hospice nurses and doctors will discontinue all medication (heart medications or breathing medications) and will begin giving morphine to "speed up" the dying process. Again, this is not true, but the answers can vary from one agency to another. Hospice is required to pay for any medications related to their terminal diagnosis.

My agency believes that we want our patients to live life to the fullest and discontinuing medications can cause a dramatic decline. We only begin pain medications and anti-anxiety medications when symptoms begin to arise. We start with the smallest doses, as we want our patients to be awake and have meaningful interactions with their family and friends."

Tracy: "What should readers be aware of when looking for a hospice program?"

Amanda: "It's important to be a smart consumer even when choosing a hospice agency. I truly recommend interviewing at least two agencies. Not all hospices are the same, and you need to ensure your goals of care are aligned with the hospice you choose. As earlier discussed, it's very important to review the medications and ensure the hospice will continue the medications.

It's also important to know how frequently a nurse and a nurse's aide will come to visit. Medicare stipulates that a nurse must see a patient at least once every two weeks. Most patients and families require more attention.

My agency has a nurse visit the first day you are ready to begin hospice. The nurse comes again the following day. So much info is given the first day, we review everything again for better retention. We also ensure all medications are in the home, as nurses frequently order additional medications if symptoms are present. We also ensure all medical equipment needed has been delivered.

From there, our nurses visit a minimum of twice a week. Another important difference is when our nurses see a patient is closer to passing away, our nurse visits daily. We also staff night nurses for any questions or needed visits/emergencies after normal business hours.

As for the nurse's aides, this can vary greatly from one agency to another. We are able to send a nurse's aide daily to assist with activities of daily living (showering, dressing, toileting, light meals prep, light house cleaning). Many agencies can only accommodate a nurse's aide once or twice a week."

Tracy: "What should people look for when researching a hospice program?"

Amanda: "When researching a hospice program, for skilled nursing facilities, look up the facilities rating on the Medicare website.* Stay away from facilities that receive only one- or two-star ratings. If they have a bed available immediately for someone on Medicaid, is it because they offer poor service? If they offer a hospice program, what hospice agencies do they work closely with and why? Drop by and take a tour of the facility. Is there a full-time medical doctor in the facility? If part time, how often is the doctor there in person? What is the facility's nurse-to-patient ratio? How many nurse's aides are on staff? Ask around about the preferred hospices. Family and friends may have had good experiences. Your physician may also have recommendations. If your loved one will be going into a facility, ask the facility which hospice they recommend. Anyone can also compare hospice agencies at Medicare.gov/hospicecompare.*

For hospice agencies offering in-home visits, how frequently do visiting nurses or nurse's aides visit? What training in pain management do they have?"

*Medicare.gov created a new website for comparing all provider types. Website: www.medicare.gov/care-compare.

Tracy: "Would you explain your Veterans Program?"

Amanda: "We honor vets: this is a broad program with many capabilities. Our team is specially trained on caring for vets specifically on PTSD, survivors' guilt, soul injury, and veteran resources. We also have a program to recognize our vets on Veterans Day. We do pinning ceremonies along with certificates. We assist with all funeral arrangements for vets and help tap into all the services they are entitled to. We honor our veterans at their passing by placing a flag over them when the funeral home or coroner picks them up from the home. We also provide the family with a flag at funeral services."

Tracy: "If someone wants to be a hospice volunteer, how do they go about applying?"

Amanda: "Anyone can volunteer for hospice. They would contact a local hospice of their choosing. We require a full background check, drug testing, and car insurance verification. From there we try to match patients and volunteers based on similar personality traits or hobbies. Some volunteers love to read books or sing to patients. Others will sit by a dying patient's side if there is no family to be with them, so patients don't die alone."

Tracy: "Would you explain the bereavement support and how it is paid for?"

Amanda: "Bereavement is not a specific service that is billed but is completely covered under the hospice benefit. Hospice services are covered by Medicare and other insurances. Essentially, hospice is given a daily rate up to a total dollar amount. Bereavement is a part of hospice services that is covered.

Bereavement can be done many different ways. There are group therapy sessions, individual counseling, over the phone conversations. We believe that bereavement begins immediately.

Many patients grieve the loss of their independence, or the loss of their health. Many grieve the loss of being the matriarch or patriarch of the family. That is part of bereavement.

Of course, the other components include the grief the family feels with the upcoming loss along with continued counseling after their passing. We have many families that have continued the bereavement counseling for years. We currently have a widow that calls our counselor when it's her husband's birthday and their wedding anniversary. There really isn't a true end point to grieving, as there are so many memories that can come flooding back with favorite songs, special dates, travel destinations, or favorite restaurants. Bereavement is always available even after 13 months."

Severe Dementia, Hospice, and Palliative Care

Usually when she reaches this stage, she will be getting palliative or hospice care. Both the Palliative-care and Hospice-care team will be able to guide you through many of these decisions. They are also a wonderful source of support.

Those diagnosed with dementia are eligible for palliative care from the time they are diagnosed. It requires a referral by her doctor. Palliative care is specialized medical care for those living with serious illnesses. The type of care provided is focused on relief from stress and symptoms of the illness. The goal of palliative care is to improve the quality of life for the patient and their family. It is a multi-pronged approach to care which includes both medical treatments and nursing, and many programs include social worker support for the caregiver.

Palliative care is not usually available for hands-on help in your home. It is usually reserved for those who have been hospitalized or having a major health crisis. Palliative care is designed to help you steer through the tough decisions.

Hospice is end-of-life care. It requires two physicians' assessments that your loved one has six months or less to life. If your loved one lasts longer than the six months, her doctor will need to write an additional order for another six months for Medicare, Medicaid, and other insurances to cover the cost of care. Hospice includes palliative care. If your loved one is in a nursing home, hospice will receive the first call in the event of a medical emergency instead of an automatic trip to the ER.

Something to be aware of, when your loved one is released from the hospital to a skilled care facility or other continuing care facility, the chain of communication can break down. As a result, you may have to stay on top of the "orders" issued by her medical care team to make sure they are communicated properly.

There is an issue with continuity of care between and within the health-care system you need to pay attention to. It will not happen every time. However, when it does, it is usually one set of doctors (within a facility or even a specialty) who do not communicate well with one another. So, if hospice or palliative care is put into place during a hospitalization, the records may not be transferred to a skilled care nursing facility.

Here is an example from my own life when I didn't know a communication breakdown occurred between medical departments. It was further complicated because I was not present at the time of my loved one's hospital discharge to confirm his release orders.

My uncle was hospitalized near the end of his life. He was being treated for prostate cancer, diabetes, and heart issues. He was released from the hospital to a rehabilitation (rehab) facility. Within hours of his arrival, he did not feel well. He called me at 4 a.m. because the facility would not send him back to the hospital. The facility staff stated, "It was against medical advice to send him back because his vital signs are stable." Seven hours later we were able to convince the facility to send him back to the hospital in an ambulance. (This meant Medicare will cover the hospitalization costs. Without the ambulance, the cost of care would have been 100 percent out-of-pocket.)

The next day he was diagnosed by his oncologist (cancer) doctor with a previously unknown cancer from his digestive tract that spread throughout his entire body and was shutting down his liver. His cancer doctor wrote orders to discontinue treatment and gave a referral for hospice care. The doctor estimated my uncle would not last longer than four weeks. His staff terminated my uncle's cancer treatment including an appointment at the hospital scheduled for that afternoon. A copy of his orders was sent to the attending physician's office to confirm diagnosis for hospice.

The attending physician never saw the cancer doctor's orders and wrote orders to release my uncle to a rehab facility the next day. My uncle moved to the rehab facility where they attempted physical therapy (PT), which he refused because he felt so ill. After PT, they sent him to the hospital for his cancer treatment. By the time I reached the rehab facility after work, my uncle was not there. I contacted the administrator in charge. They sent him to his cancer appointment per the hospital discharge orders. No matter how many times I explained the situation to the administrator, she could not deviate from the orders they received from the hospital. Fifteen minutes after I arrived my uncle was returned to the facility where the driver explained to the facility administrator the appointment had been cancelled and that he was supposed to be in hospice care.

The administrator explained to me that they were a rehab only facility. We were given one week to find hospice care, since that was the length of time Medicare would pay for his stay without him participating in the prescribed rehabilitation program. After that week if he had not moved, he would be converted to a private pay patient at the cost of $12,000 to $15,000 per month depending on his care needs.

It is not easy to find hospice care without a nurse navigator or social worker. Because of the mix-up, a nurse navigator or social worker was not available to us.

However, one of the nurse navigators from the hospital took pity on us and gave me a list of the hospice facilities in the area that were approved by Medicare. I was told there was no space available at each facility I contacted. There was nowhere for him to go. For better or worse, my uncle passed on day seven—his last day at the facility covered by Medicare.

Had I been at the hospital at the time of his release, I would have caught the error on the discharge orders. The hospital staff would have directed him to a hospice facility. He would not have gone through the duress of being forced into physical and occupational therapy he did not need. It would not have extended his life, but it would have made him more comfortable during his last week. It would also have reduced the stress on myself and the rest of the family trying to find him an available space when we should have been focused on his care and comfort.

If available, hospital social workers and nurse navigators will help you find placement quickly, because they are pressured by hospitals to get the patient discharged. They know which facilities have beds available on the day the person leaves. However, the beds fill fast, and you cannot wait more than the day before the space is no longer available, as I discovered. Planning ahead and getting on wait lists gives you options when the time comes. By planning ahead, you may not have a choice but to take the space that is immediately available for the short term but stay on the list for your preferred location. This means you can make the move to the preferred facility when a bed become available.

For better or for worse, whoever is her health care power of attorney will need to stay on top of the medical records and doctors' orders. This may result in repeated requests and consultations with her medical care team to get copies. It is worth the effort to save you the grief. Having a copy of the correct orders will give you leverage with the care facility.

Additionally, when your loved one is actively dying, they may be in pain. If that is the case, you will need to stay on top of their pain medication. For example, Michelle, whose name has been changed to protect her family's privacy, shared her experience with her father's death and pain medication being withheld for administrative reasons.

> *Even when Hospice is involved, it's really important to stay on top of the loved one's pain needs. My dad was on morphine and staff were anal about making sure he didn't get it any sooner than the prescribed time.*
>
> *Pain meds were an issue because of the dispensing policy in the facility. It was restricted to nursing staff. If they were taking care of other patients, it meant hunting them down. Then they had to review the chart, look at the notes and the prescription, and get the meds from a locked cabinet. And meanwhile my dad was in a lot of pain.*

One of the ways that may help reduce this issue is to make sure your loved one's doctor prescribes the pain medication as "scheduled medication on a four-hour basis," not as needed, also known as "PRN," (Latin for "pro re nata," meaning "as the thing is needed"). There are no guarantees, but it may help.

What are your feelings about the location of where your loved one's death will happen?

Your loved one may have expressed a wish to die at home. This might not be possible. Most people with dementia pass in hospitals and nursing homes.

Some families choose to bring their family member home from the hospital or nursing home at the end of their life. They may do so with or without support from hospice. Home care is very difficult especially because it involves dispensing pain medications—usually every four hours. Bringing family members home is not very common.

Some families expect to care for their family member at home until an emergency, like a fall or low-blood-sugar-induced coma or stroke tosses those plans out the window. In the last three months of life, repeated hospitalizations will be unpleasant for her and stressful for you with all the ups and downs. On a side note, if your loved one is admitted to the hospital more than once in a 30-day period for the same issue, Medicare looks at this as a readmission and will penalize the hospital for releasing the patient too soon. At the time of this writing, if that is the case, the hospital will pick up the tab for the "readmit."

Some families may have strong aversions to death in their homes and will do anything to avoid it. Other families may be guided by religious or cultural preferences for the chosen location.

It's a good idea to consider early on where you want the death to happen. There is a serious bed shortage for this kind of care in the United States, so you may find it as difficult, as I did, in finding an available bed in a nursing home or a hospice program. Keep in mind, not everyone is approved for hospice – depending on what kind of hospice programs are available or if the prescribing doctors don't agree. Consider contacting fellow support group participants, social workers, and the clergy because they are also good resources for navigating the system.

If your loved one is on Medicaid, there can be a year or more wait list for an available bed, even in a nursing home. If a bed becomes available before your loved one needs it, let the facility know. They can move your loved one's name down on their list so the bed can go to someone else who

> Group homes care for one to six residents, have one to two 24-hour caregivers who are trained medical technician and oversee the activities of daily living (ADL). Hospice agencies supply trained nurses and nurse's aides for in-home end-of-life care.

could use it. That said, it is not uncommon for someone on Medicaid who is dying to end up in the hospital, at which point a Social Worker will make arrangements for their care at a skilled nursing facility or an adult family home, also known as group homes or board and care homes.

It is also important to know in advance whom to contact when the death occurs. If hospice is involved, they will take care of the details for you. Skilled care nursing facilities will do the same. If your loved one plans to die at home, contact her primary care doctor to discuss what advanced arrangements are needed.

If she dies from natural causes at home and you choose to call 9-1-1, the emergency medical technician may attempt to resuscitate your loved one, unless you have a DNR order (Do Not Resuscitate) on hand. It is their job. Keep in mind the police may investigate the death.

If you have made arrangements with a funeral home, they will transport your loved one and fill out the death certificate in addition to funeral arrangements.

While it is important for the death of your loved one to be certified by medical personnel soon after passing, you may invite family members or clergy in to take some time with your loved one's body before it is removed. Not everyone will want to do this, but it may give you some closure.

Death with Dignity

Your loved one may express a wish to die with dignity, also known as physician-assisted dying or physician-assisted suicide. At the time of this writing, in nine states it means the terminally ill may seek to end their life with lethal doses of medication prescribed by their physician. In order to qualify, the person must be terminally ill and in their right state of mind. In states that do not allow the use of medications, this means your loved one will stop eating. There can be many reasons someone who is terminally ill may wish control over their own death, physical and emotional pain being the main reason.

At the time of this writing, the states with Death with Dignity laws on their books are:

California	New Jersey
Colorado	Oregon
District of Columbia	Vermont
Hawaii	Washington
Maine	

In 2009, Montana's Supreme Court declared Physician-Assisted Suicide (PAS) consistent with Montana's statutes and constitution, but the legislature has not passed any legislation further defining the terms or requirements.[79]

In someone with dementia, especially Alzheimer's disease, deciding to stop eating is usually the route they choose.

For example, Becky, whose name has been changed to protect her family's privacy, shared her experience with her father's death with dignity.

> *My dad had had a stroke. He was suffering from old age dementia. And he was with it enough that he asked for a gun. We ended up allowing him to die with dignity. Hospice came in and he got morphine to help with the pain along with any food or liquids he wanted. He stopped eating solids and in the days before his death, he rarely ate anything. I remember a couple of times he had some pudding. Most of the time the staff gave him these sponges that helped keep his mouth moist and I recall he'd have sips of water or ice chips. It was a tough place to be in, but we respected his right to determine his future.*

Death with dignity is a very personal and emotional decision. To learn more about death with dignity visit Death with Dignity's website www.deathwithdignity.org. Not everyone will choose this path. Not everyone will agree with the decision because of moral or religious beliefs. You need to be aware that this topic may come up in end-of-life conversations, so you are better prepared emotionally to deal with the subject.

* * *

This journey with dementia is hard. Many things will not go as planned. You will run the emotional gamut: anger, compassion, fear, guilt, joy, and even face your own mortality. Give yourself the emotional space you need to cope with each challenge. Continue to take care of yourself. This is not a journey that should be taken alone.

Accept any help that is offered to you during this time. Make time for yourself to decompress, release your guilt and anger. Use the reframing technique, breathing exercises, and short quick walks, see Self Care in *Distraction Techniques* page 132. Take time to talk to others, whether in a support group, or with a counselor, social worker, or a member of the clergy. Do not beat yourself up or punish yourself; instead, choose to recognize you are worth the effort to maintain your health and live.

Through each stage of dementia, the writing becomes clearer on the blackboard. You cannot change the outcome. You are doing everything you can. You can choose how you will cope.

Recognize that each emotional experience is like a grain of sand in an oyster. With help and healing, the experience that was once an irritation, trial, or loss can grow in luster and beauty giving you benefits you never imagined: the ability to teach others how to survive the caregiving journey; bonding deeply with other caregivers; building strong, life-long emotional connections and support.

When you've reached the end of this journey, embrace your grief—it is filled with many valuable lessons and you will be stronger for it. Then mine for *your* pearl. List all the benefits from your experience, and what you've learned. Share the positives of your experience with others. Let it be a beacon in the dark guiding other caregivers to safety like seafarers following the stars.

"I will love the light for it shows me the way, yet I will endure the darkness because it shows me the stars." ~Og Mandino

Chapter 18: Long-Term Care Options

"Always do whatever's next." ~George Carlin

There are many reasons a family cannot take care of their loved one at home, even with help. There are many reasons someone with dementia may need to be moved to a nursing home or other residential care facility. For example, when the primary caregiver becomes ill or is too worn down to give good care; or other demands, including caring for children, or a spouse; or a job that makes it impossible for someone to be a full-time caregiver. Another common reason is the person with dementia has medical needs that are more complex than the caregiver is able or qualified to handle.

It's also very common that caregivers wait too long to place a family member in a long-term care facility. It makes sense that you and your loved one should discuss long-term care before it is needed, so that when the time comes, he will have time to adjust to the new living situation. It can take from three to six months or longer for a person with dementia to adjust to a new living environment.

Putting your loved one in a nursing home or other care facility can be a very tough decision to make. A time may come when placing your loved one in a skilled nursing facility is the best decision for their well-being and yours, especially if you cannot manage their behaviors. If he is physically aggressive, a skilled nursing facility may be the only safe option.

There are a number of other care options to be considered. They range from the minimal support of assisted living, where couples can live together, to settings with full time care.

Paying for Care

It is not uncommon for family members to disagree about plans for long-term care. The family could be divided over whether he should stay at home or be moved to some level of skilled nursing facility. It is helpful if all the involved members of the family discuss this early in the diagnosis. Disagreements and misunderstandings are often caused when not everyone has all of the facts and their perception about the current situation does not align with the reality.

Here are things to consider before having a family meeting. <u>First, there are not enough dementia care facilities available for those with dementia.</u> If you find a facility you like, get on the waiting list well ahead of time. If you delay until your loved one needs to find a place quickly, such as after a hospital stay, you will have to take whatever is available at the time. The facility may not offer the quality of care you are looking for. If you are on the wait list for a facility, and a bed becomes available, you may change to the facility of your choice.

There are no public monies designated to help with this cost. Most families cover the cost from their loved one's resources such as pensions or assets, for example their home and investments. Medicare only pays for short periods of time, usually less than 90 days, after a hospitalization for the treatment of a serious illness or injury.

Finding a facility takes time, especially if there is no long-term care insurance or if someone is on Medicaid. Medicaid only pays for care for those who cannot afford to pay for it. Medicaid beds are few and can take up to a year or longer to become available. If this is your situation, get on waiting lists a year or more before you need this service.

Due to the high cost of care, those from the middle class will deplete their assets in a very short period of time and end up on Medicaid. Because the federal and state regulations are so restrictive, if one spouse needs care and the other is healthy, only a small stipend will be available for the spouse who continues to live at home. If you choose divorce as a financial option, you will no longer have power of attorney for your loved one. Consult an attorney prior to making any decisions. It is very important to plan well in advance for possible ways to pay for long-term care.

Keep in mind that long-term care insurance policies will help pay for part of the cost of care in the home. Some policies only pay for specific types of care facilities and may have certain exclusions. Most will only pay a portion of the cost of daily care. While long-term care insurance does help, there will still be a need to look at other sources of funding.

In 2018, nursing home care averaged $89,000 per year, with the cost in Alaska significantly higher. The cost of assisted living ranged from $39,600 in the southern and plains states to upwards of $72,000 in the Northeast and West Coast.[80]

Types of Care Facilities

There are many different types of care facilities, ranging from continuing care at home to skilled nursing facilities. When considering a facility, make sure they can provide the level of care your loved one needs. Here is a brief overview of available options:

Continuing Care at Home. These programs are modeled after continuing care retirement communities. There is an administrative fee paid up front, then a monthly fee which guarantees there is care for the rest of the person's life. This service takes place in your loved one's home instead of in a facility. The services go from meals only up to twenty-four-hour supervision. For example, Springpoint Choice, a New Jersey-based nonprofit provider, or Fedelta Home Care based in Washington State.

There is also a new emerging at-home care model by a North Carolina company called CarePods.[81] Their members are seniors who live within a 15-mile radius and are grouped into small, member pods. Each pod is overseen by a dedicated registered nurse case manager who helps coordinate their members clinical needs, which includes medication education, scheduling doctor's appointments, in addition to other services.

Adult Family Homes. Not all adult family homes provide dementia care. Those that do, provide fewer services than a nursing home. They are not covered by Medicare or Medicaid. They provide a room, meals, supervision, and some additional services.

Assisted Living Facilities. They supply a room, meals, activities, help with tasks like bathing, dressing, eating, and supervision. In general, they do not provide nursing services or medical care. Their residents must be able to walk and can help take care of themselves. Depending on the facility, some specialize in caring for those with dementia, while others do not. Some may supervise medications or even have limited medical care available during the daytime within the facility. However, they may discharge anyone who is unable to walk, needs regular nursing care, or behaves in a disruptive or dangerous manner. <u>As with all facilities, those who have regular visits from family and friends will get better care.</u>

Continuing Care Retirement Facilities. These facilities supply a range of care from independent living through long-term care in a campus style facility. The idea is when someone moves in, they are healthy. Depending on the facility, they may initially provide meals as part of the basic package. If a resident's health declines, then he will be moved to the part of the facility with the level of care that matches his needs. This may be assisted living or skilled nursing. Keep in mind that not all facilities can accommodate dementia care. These facilities require a down payment and/or an entrance fee along with a monthly fee. A deposit is often needed to get on the wait list.

Depending on the facility set-up, the property may supply rental units or condominiums. In a condominium, the resident pays a mortgage plus fees which pay for services such as building maintenance, yard care, recreational facilities, security systems, and transportation to local shopping. For a person with limited income who has dementia, there might be state programs available to cover some of the cost for long-term care in this type of facility.

Some couples choose to move to such a facility so they may stay together because of the options for assistance. However, not all continuing care facilities will accept someone with dementia. Running out of money is a deciding factor depending on the type of community. If the community is a not-for-profit, once the couple is accepted, they will be cared for even if they run out of money. If the community is for profit, however, they may be asked to leave when they run out of money.

Before deciding on a continuing care retirement facility, confirm they are accredited by the Continuing Care Accreditation Commission. Their website is www.carf.org. Just because a facility is accredited, does not mean they are able to take care of someone with dementia. Ask the following:

- If they are not accredited, ask what kind of state or industry certifications do they have?
- How often are they inspected and by whom?
- If a resident decides not to stay, are the entrance fees or deposit refundable?
- Will someone with dementia be asked to leave? What if the dementia was unknown to be pre-existing at the time of admission, will they be asked to leave?
- Are there any additional entrance fees or monthly fees for someone with dementia?
- What other reasons could a person or couple be asked to leave?
- What services and activities does the monthly fee cover?
- Is participation in group meals or group activities required? If yes, what are the penalties for not participating? What if someone does not like the food, what are their options? Will they accommodate food allergies? Do they have vegetarian or vegan options?
- Do they have enough assisted living spaces available for immediate move in?
- Do they have a skilled nursing unit?
    - Does the nursing unit accept people with dementia?
    - If yes, when you saw it during the tour, did you like the feel of the nursing unit?
    - How are medical needs being met in the nursing unit? Who provides that medical care? How is the medical care supervised?
    - Are you satisfied with the quality of available care in the nursing unit?
- How are other medical, dental, and vision needs taken care of? Do they have their own doctors on staff?
    - If yes, are all residents required to use this doctor?
    - If yes, will you have to change health insurances providers to cover the cost of the medical staff visits?

- Is a physical exam required as part of the admission process?
- Do the doctors on staff have experience with geriatric care? Do they understand the medical needs of someone with dementia?
- If there are no doctors on staff, what happens in the event of an emergency?
- If there are no medical facilities available onsite, is transportation to medical appointments provided?
- Will their entrance fee or any portion of it be returned to their estate if someone passes before all the money is spent on care?
- What happens to your investment if the facility goes bankrupt?

Check with your state's consumer protection office or the office of your state's attorney general for any complaints filed against the facility. Read the facilities policies and the quality of care they provide before investing your money.

Nursing Homes. The term nursing homes, also known as skilled nursing facilities (SNF), stirs up bad images in many people's minds. However, these facilities generally give good care. They may also be the best choice for a person who has dementia. SNFs take people who are ill and need specific medical care such as assistance with feeding or feeding tubes. They may also accept people who are less ill or disabled, often people who are discharged from hospitals.

The SNF may or may not be certified for Medicare and/or Medicaid payments for care. Not all SNFs accept Medicare or Medicaid. Medicare only covers patients with serious conditions that need skilled nursing for a short time period, usually 90 days or less.

When considering a SNF for your loved one:
- Check to make sure they accept either Medicare or Medicaid
- If your loved one is accepted at one level of care (and payment type), will he be able to stay if his care needs increase, or the source of funding changes from personal resources and insurance to Medicaid?
- If the SNF accepts Medicare and/or Medicaid, is it licensed?
- Is it inspected by the state?
- Being inspected by the state does not guarantee the SNF meets the standards. Ask to look at their most recent inspection report. It will list any deficiencies. How are they addressing the deficiencies?
- Are they a memory care facility? Do they offer programs designed for those with dementia?
- Are there regularly scheduled activities someone with dementia would enjoy participating in?

- Does the care cost more because of dementia? Increased cost does not always mean better care

- Is it a private pay only facility? Can you or your loved one afford it? If your loved one goes on Medicaid down the road, will he be asked to leave?

- Is the SNF close enough that family members and friends will visit? Visiting family members mean better care for your loved one, especially if they stay in touch with the staff, and it will be better for his overall well-being

- Will he be moved to a different unit when his dementia increases? If yes, will it be within the same facility or to a different facility? Do you like the unit he would be sent to?

- How much medication will be used to control behavior? Often better care from the staff and having enough staff means your loved one will need less medication. **Understaffed facilities use behavior-controlling medication to compensate for staffing issues**

Companies like *A Place for Mom* offer a check list to rate SNF facilities. They and other similar services offer help in narrowing down the area facilities based on your loved one's needs. They are paid by the SNF facility if your loved one moves in.

If the SNF accepts Medicare, you can search through Medicare's website to view and compare SNFs in your area. The link is www.medicare.gov/care-compare. The website uses a five-star rating system to help you compare nursing homes. No rating system is perfect, and not every facility gets a five-star grade. Also, the system does not specifically address dementia care or how easy it will be to visit your loved one in their facility. Use the rating system, but don't make it the only criteria you use for choosing a facility. You should always visit a SNF in person before making a decision.

Signs of a Bad Nursing Home

If you have never been in a nursing home, how do you know what to look for? The following questions have been adapted from AARP's warning signs for bad nursing homes.

1. What does it smell like? Is there a strong odor from urine or feces or a heavy smell of disinfectant used to cover up odors? This is an indication there may not be enough staff to help residents to the bathroom.

2. How clean is the facility? The best way to check is to ask if you can view a resident's room.

3. Is there a lack of privacy? Are residents being undressed in private? Are they being dressed in the hallway? Is the staff knocking on doors before entering rooms?

4. Are the residents treated respectfully? Does the staff know the resident's name? Or do they call them by a nickname like "love," "honey," "mamma," "papa" or "sweetie"? Does the staff speak to them respectfully or rudely?

5. Are there unanswered calls for help? How long does it take for a resident to get care after pushing a call button?

6. Are there appropriate grab bars in bathrooms and other safety equipment? Are there handrails in the hallways?

7. Is there evident loneliness or inactivity among the residents? Are the residents parked in chairs around the facility by themselves or left sitting in a wheelchair in a hallway? Do they look lonely or unhappy?

8. Is there enough staff to help with eating? A resident should not be sitting with a full plate of food in front of them if they can't feed themselves without help.

9. Do staff members acknowledge you or is your presence ignored?

10. Is there a big difference between how well furnished and lit the main entrance and common areas are when compared to the residents' rooms and hallways?

11. Are restraints used? You should not see any restraints in a nursing home, as they are no longer allowed. Quality nursing homes choose respectful and safe ways to prevent falls and wandering. For example, residents who are wheelchair bound may use lap buddies, a foam pad placed across the lap and tucked under the arms of the wheelchair to prevent falls, but the staff do not leave those residents sitting alone in the hallway. They address wandering by redirecting residents to an activity suited to their skill level, such as singing, simple art projects, or storytelling.

Here is an example from my own life with regards to care facilities. Both of my parents and my uncle were asked to leave several different facilities for various reasons, leaving us very little time to find a place for them to stay. Sometimes, we were not successful.

My father was asked to leave five different care facilities because they were not equipped to handle his behavioral issues, which included escaping, or Medicaid would only pay for three days of his stay based on the type of care at a specific facility. I was able to move him in with me and my husband after he was evicted from the fifth facility. Because I did not have power of attorney, I had to convince a few family members, who felt I might not be able to handle the caregiving, to give their blessings. My father wasn't ready for skilled care at that point. His behavior was the only way he could communicate his needs as the dementia strengthened its hold.

On a separate note, once your loved one transitions to a SNF memory care unit, it is common for you to have mixed emotions about visiting the facility. Knowing how to visit a nursing home helps you and your loved one, because patients who have family members that visit regularly get better care. For strategies on visiting a nursing home, see the blog post: *How to Visit a Nursing Home*, on my website

tracycramperkins.com/blog.

The Department of Veterans Affairs (VA)

The VA is required to take care of people with service-related illnesses first. After that the VA assists other veterans based on available space and services. The treatment options available in one area may not be available in another. A veteran with dementia might be admitted to a VA long-term care hospital or even a contracted nursing home, only to be discharged later. A few VA facilities even offer respite and/or family support, but the policies differ between VA hospitals. If you are having difficulties getting help from the VA, contact www.caregiver.va.gov first. You can also speak with a VA Care Ombudsman during normal office hours at most VA hospitals and clinics.

* * *

Another excellent resource, available for free, is AARP's *Prepare To Care* guide, accessible online at:

https://www.aarp.org/content/dam/aarp/home-and-family/caregiving/2012-10/PrepareToCare-Guide-FINAL.pdf. There is an in-depth section at the end of the guide which includes a place to list your loved one's legal, financial, and medical contacts with spaces for medications, their Medicare information, and VA Benefits. It also includes a section for which bills are due and when, passwords, and other information you will need for your situation.

Now you know there are options available for you when you need the help. Start looking for the next level of facilities at least a year before you need them. Where your loved one is in his dementia journey will help you determine how to prepare for whatever's next.

Chapter 19: The Signs that Death is Approaching

What's Covered in This Chapter
- The Signals of Active Dying
- Dealing with the Days and Moments before Death
- The Moment of Death
- Death and Emotional Healing

It is difficult to predict the moment of death no matter what the cause. However, there are certain signals associated with the body shutting down that can give us a general time frame such as days or weeks. The signals may vary in their order from one person to another.

In the last six months of life, there is generally a diagnosis of other conditions such as kidney failure or congestive heart failure. There will also be an increase in trips to the hospital — both emergency room admissions and hospital stays.

In the last two to three months, speech will be limited to six words a day or less. There will be increased difficulty swallowing. You will notice more choking on food or liquids. They will be unable to sit upright or walk without help. They will need adult diapers for total incontinence. The likelihood of pneumonia increases.

Each person's death is unique. While some people will show clear signs of dying, in others the signs will be hard to spot and still others may not show any signs at all. If you see one or two of the following signs, it might not mean death is near. But it is important to let your loved one's medical care team, palliative care team, or hospice care team know. They can give you more information about what the signals mean and what to expect. For the rest of this chapter they will be referred to as the medical care team.

The Signals of Active Dying [82]

Loss of Appetite

A month or so before dying, your loved one may stop eating hard-to-digest foods such as meat. At this point she will only accept bland foods as her need for energy dwindles. Eventually she will resist or refuse meals and liquids. A person with severe dementia may no longer be able to swallow.

Once active dying begins, hydration and tube feeding become an issue for the person. Standard practice at this stage is hydration by hand, either using ice chips to suck on, moist swabs, or water from a dropper. This will relieve dry mouth.

Excess Fatigue and Sleep

It is common at this point for the person to sleep most of the day and night. Her metabolism is slowing. The lack of food and water leads to dehydration. This type of dehydration releases brain chemicals, such as endorphins, which reduces pain and discomfort. At this point, it becomes difficult to wake her. Her awareness of what is going on around her will begin to fade.

Physical Weakness

She will be unable to sit up without assistance. Moving in bed and even lifting her arms and head become harder.

Mental Confusion

In the final weeks, she may speak to people who aren't visible in the room, such as seeing her parents. She may talk about seeing a favorite travel location or other people who are living or dead. The disorientation of this stage may be difficult to determine if she is in the late stages of dementia, because she may have been behaving this way for a long time.

A few days before fully receding there may be a moment of lucidity, where she appears to be in her right mind. It can last from less than an hour up to a full day where she may share some final words.

Social Withdrawal

This can be caused by reduced blood flow and oxygen to the brain. She is preparing for death. Speak to her calmly and directly. You don't need to speak loudly or shake her awake to talk to her. Assure her you are there for her. She is aware and may be able to hear but is losing her ability to respond. Reassure her that her life was meaningful, and the family will be well cared for when she is gone. Thank her for the time she spent with you, that you love her, and let her know it is okay to go.

Labored Breathing

Changes in breathing become more pronounced. Her breathing may become shallower, shift speeds between rapid and slow, and may make rattling or gurgling sounds (death rattles). Changes in her heart rate may alter her breathing. She may take several deep breaths followed by longer pauses before resuming regular breathing (Cheyne-Stokes breathing). This can be very difficult for family members while they wait for her last breath. In the last 24-hours her blood oxygen levels will drop. The loss of oxygen may cause her eyes to change color.

Breathing might be easier when sitting up with extra support or when lying on her side with pillows under her head and behind her back. It's tough to listen to labored breathing, but it does not generally cause her any extra pain. Sometimes the use of oxygen can help and using a cool mist humidifier to add moisture to the air may add some comfort and relief.

Changes in Urination

Darkened urine and decreased urination happen because she is drinking less fluids and her kidneys are shutting down. Sometimes a catheter might be used to prevent blockages. If needed, your health care team will give you instructions for taking care of the catheter.

Swelling of the Feet, Hands, and Ankles

Her kidneys are shutting down and body fluids are no longer being filtered the way they used to. This type of swelling is caused by low protein. Remember, she stopped eating meat. The stored body fluids show up in the areas below the heart like the feet, hand, and ankles. The hips may show some swelling too. This can also happen if the medical care team gives IV fluids to ease discomfort.

Blotchy Skin Tones

The skin becomes blotchy, becoming darker and has a gray or bluish color. This is also known as 'mottled.' It shows the most on the backside of the body and in the arms and legs. This happens because the blood circulation is slowing down in the body.

Cool or Hot Fingers and Toes

In addition to changes in the skin's color, the fingers and toes feel cool to the touch, at other times they may feel hot and clammy. She may not actually feel the cold. Extra blankets can be used for warmth, if it will make you feel better. Do not use electric blankets because at this stage the electric blanket can burn the skin and too many blankets may cause her to become hot and restless.

Changes in Vision

She may turn her head and look directly at a light source, such as a table lamp, ceiling light or wall sconce. This is due to loss of eyesight. Make sure any lighting in the room she is in is soft, indirect lighting to help her see better.

Muscles Twitch

Quick, involuntary muscle twitches are called myoclonic jerks. Combined with the loss of reflexes in the arms and legs, it is another signal death is approaching. While it is not painful, it can be very disturbing to watch her out-of-control twitching. There are medications that can reduce the twitch and improve sleep. Check with the medical care team.

Difficulty Controlling Pain

It is important to give her the pain medication as prescribed by her medical care team. If you notice the medication does not seem to be working or is having concerning side effects, contact her medical care team. Alternative pain management methods, such as music therapy, massage, and relaxation routines, including laughter, may be used with medications to reduce anxiety and discomfort.

Dealing with the Days and Moments before Death

Hindsight is a big bully carrying a Louisville Slugger baseball bat. Second guessing each decision you make regarding end-of-life care gives hindsight the opportunity to hit you out of the ball park and into the minivan's windshield. End-of-life care is always harder than you think, even when you are prepared. You might wonder if withholding a feeding tube is the right decision for your loved one, even though your medical care team tells you that it won't prevent or delay her death. Or if you should choose not to honor her signed Do Not Resuscitate (DNR) order, would that be the right thing to do?[83]

Your emotions will run you through everything you "should have done." It's hard not to second guess yourself. Consider this: because you are thinking about what you should do means you are assessing all aspects of her care, including her express wishes. That alone should reassure you that you have made the best decisions you could with the information you have at the time.[84]

End-of-life decisions are some of the hardest decisions you will ever have to make. Those who specialize in end-of-life-care, such as hospice, can explain the options with each decision. They can show you that the decisions you are making will not speed up your loved one's death, nor will it prolong her life. Rely on their expertise to help you make decisions so you don't become overwhelmed. Use your loved one's wishes, if she recorded them when she was able to make her wishes known, as your guide.

It is also important to know in advance whom to contact when the death occurs. If hospice is involved, they will take care of the details for you. Skilled care nursing facilities will do the same.

If your loved one will die at home, contact her primary care doctor prior to her passing to discuss arrangements. If she dies from natural causes at home and you choose to call 9-1-1, the emergency medical technician may attempt to resuscitate her, unless you have a DNR Order (Do Not Resuscitate also known as a P.O.L.S.T.) on hand. It is their job. Keep in mind if you call 9-1-1, the police may investigate the death.

If you have made arrangements with a funeral home, they will transport your loved one and fill out the death certificate in addition to funeral arrangements.

After your loved one passes, you may not know what to do next. You may be numb with grief and exhaustion; small details will slip through the cracks. The chapter, *When Your Caregiving Responsibilities are Over*, details the steps to take and whom to contact. Prepare those steps in advance of your loved one's passing so you won't get clobbered with more than you can handle. And put that Louisville Slugger back in the closet where it belongs.

The Moment of Death

Your self-worth should not be measured by whether you were with your loved one at the moment of death but by the strength of your relationship over a lifetime. Death is unpredictable. It is not always possible to be present at the moment of death. You can stay by your loved one's side for hours, then take a moment to use the bathroom. When you return to her side, she is gone. Perhaps she wanted to spare you the pain of being present for the finale. Or she could hang on for a specific person to arrive or something in particular to be said like "I love you," "I forgive you," or "Please forgive me." Blaming yourself because you "weren't there" or feeling cheated by missing the final moment is setting yourself up for unnecessary guilt. We carry enough emotional baggage in our lifetime, so don't add this to the pile.

Remember the importance of touch. Touch is a way to tell your loved one you are there. It shares affection and comfort and brings calm for you and your loved one. Touch can penetrate the fog that is dementia in those final hours, letting them know they are not forgotten and alone. That they have value. The important thing is finding out what type of touch is meaningful to your loved one. When you are unsure what to do for them, hold their hand, caress their cheek or hair, or put your hand on their arm or shoulder.

Sometimes this simple act isn't so much for your loved one as it is for the rest of the family. We are so insulated from death these days that we don't know what to do. By showing your family your compassion, they are more likely to do the same thing. If your loved one, who may be in a semi-conscious stupor, responds to your touch—even with a single tear, the power of that connection will be with you for a lifetime.

Death and Emotional Healing

Death is the beginning of healing. It is quite normal to feel relief once your loved one passes. They have been released from the damages of an awful disease. Hindsight will insist you feel guilty. Instead, it is time to grieve, to remember, and laugh through the tears.

Canadian mystery writer, Louise Penny, shared with her fans her caregiving journey with her husband, Michael, during his battle with Alzheimer's Disease. With her permission, here is an excerpt from her newsletter on her final night with her husband, after the rest of the family said their goodbyes for the night. She described the last moments she spent with her husband, their dog, Bishop, and the hospice doctor:

But that night was mine. Just the three of us. Michael and Bishop and me.

I set up an easy chair by his hospital bed, and a little table, and sat there while he slept, Bishop at my feet.

Later that evening it was clear something had changed. His breathing was more laboured.

I called Dr. Giannangelo (again) and interrupted her dinner. Again, absolutely no complaint, just: I'll be right there.

And she was.

As she prepared the medications, I held Michael and whispered prayers. All the prayers I could think of. Serenity Prayer, Third Step Prayer, Lord's Prayer. Now I lay me down to sleep…. And the Prayer of St Francis. Michael's favourite prayer. The one he recited from memory at a candlelight vigil as we held hands with neighbours, after 9/11.

It seemed to calm him. I know for sure it calmed me.

Then Dr. Giannangelo and I administered the syringes.

I whispered to Michael, over and over: God loves you. I love you. You are kind and brave and handsome and loved. We are all so proud of you. I'm so happy to be your wife. God loves you. I love you. You can let go.

Over and over.

Dr. Giannangelo had to go back to her office, briefly, for something. I walked her to the door.

And when I returned to the bedroom, Michael was gone. In the twinkling of an eye.

He was so peaceful, so serene, so relaxed. His eyes closed, his body at rest. I think I just sighed.

He was across the finish line.

Losing someone you love is very difficult. Losing someone you love to dementia is long and agonizing. You choose how you will experience your loved one's death. I hope in your grief you choose love and relief over guilt and pain.

Chapter 20: Digital Estates and How to Deactivate a Loved One's Social Media, Email Accounts, and Other Digital Estates

Digital Estates

Digital Estates (DE) are electronic information assets that exist on the internet or other devices and are less readily and tangibly transferable than your mother's jewelry. Working with Digital Estates (DE) is a relatively new concept. We are spending more of our lives online with social media, banking, shopping, sending emails, reading books, streaming content, and playing games. At the time of this writing very few states have laws governing DE. I am not an attorney, and in no way is this intended to take the place of legal advice. However, your loved one needs to consider the effects on their DE upon their passing. If your loved one dies without planning for their DE it will be difficult for their heirs to access their bank accounts, deactivate social media, or take care of their wishes.

They will need to create a DE document, known as a Master Password List, which lists all of the websites they visit on a daily, weekly, monthly, or on an annual basis. For example:

- Banking
- Investment accounts
- Insurance policies
- Social media
- Email
- Blog
- Other online services, for example:
    - Video and music streaming services
    - Online shopping
    - Online payment services and cryptocurrency

Include the websites, their usernames, security challenge information, and passwords. You may be able to figure out their passwords, but you may not know her favorite bull mastiff Brutus's third middle name was Lemon Drop. Like a letter of instructions, it is not a legal document and should not be included in the will. The will is a public document and is released to the public upon passing during probate. Instead, specify in the will where the document is kept, or share the location with a trusted relative or friend. Because passwords are changed regularly, make sure the Master Password List is up to date at least quarterly. Include in the document the date it was revised.

Keep in mind if your loved one uses a password app, they will need to read the Terms of Service (TOS) to make sure their heirs can access the passwords. Generally speaking, the safest way to guarantee heirs have access to accounts, without having to jump through legal hoops, is to create a Master Password List.

Deactivating Social Media

Now here's the painful part, the rules governing what happens to social media accounts after death are spelled out in the Terms of Service and vary by service provider. Many social media sites offer added service that can be used to deactivate an account or in some instances create a temporary memorial.

The following are examples of how to find the instructions for deactivating social media accounts of Facebook, Twitter, and Google (which owns Twitter) and their policies for deactivating social media. As with all social media, it will change based on new Federal Regulations and unforeseen circumstances, so included here are the search terms you will need to locate each company's policies.

Facebook

Logon to Facebook via your own account, in the upper right-hand corner of the screen click on the account icon then select Help & Support in the dropdown menu. Click on the Help Center icon. Enter the search terms "remove deceased family member's account." You will be directed to their page stating the policy with step-by-step instructions to deactivate the account.

At the time of this writing, Facebook requires the following to prove your claim as an immediate family member or executor of their estate:

- A copy of the deceased's death certificate. If you do not have the death certificate you will need to prove your claim with at least one of the following documents
  - Power of attorney
  - Birth certificate of the deceased
  - Last will and testament
  - Estate letter

Without the death certificate, they will require one of the following:

- Obituary notice

- Memorial card

This must match the information they have on file for your loved one. Never send personal information such as a Social Security number.

Twitter

Logon to Twitter via your own account, click on the Terms of Service link at the bottom of the screen. Select Twitter Rules and Policies. Enter the search terms "deceased user." You will be directed to Twitter's page stating their policy with instructions to contact them.

Once Twitter receives your request, they will ask for documentation to prove you are authorized to act on the behalf of the deceased, they will send you an email with instructions to provide the following information to prove your claim:

- Information about the deceased
- A copy of your ID
- A copy of the deceased's death certificate

Google

Google uses Inactive Account Manager (IAM) which allows your loved one to assign up to 10 trusted friends or relatives as beneficiaries of their online accounts. Conveniently, anyone can Google "Inactive Account Manager" and Google will direct you to the IAM page.

In IAM, they can specify what they want to happen for each Google service they use. If they use IAM they will list a specified period of time for Google to monitor for inactivity in their account. The IAM allows them to create emails which will be sent to their contacts once the time period they specify has elapsed. If they specify in the settings, the service will allow their contacts to download data from the accounts. If they set up this feature, they will need their contacts' mobile phone numbers to ensure their contacts can download their data with an access code sent to their phone once they click on the download link in the email.

No emails will be sent to their contacts while they are setting up the account. The contacts will not know they have set up this service unless your loved one alerted them ahead of time or the time period on the account has elapsed and they receive the email. Remember to update your IAM account when someone changes their email account, cell phone number, or passes away.

What Happens to Email Accounts?

Just like with social media accounts, they will need to read the TOS for each of their email accounts to find out what happens to it when they pass. In most cases, the TOS gives a nontransferable license. Which means nobody can access their email once they die. Some service providers consider the account terminated upon their death. Federal law does not allow email service providers to share the contents of emails without a court order or a consent from the individual who uses the account. If they want their heirs to have access to their email after they pass, they will need to write a statement granting them access and include it with their will.

What Happens to Financial Accounts?

Some financial institutions will allow people to specify their beneficiaries through their website. They may also state their preferences directly with the banking institution when they open or update their account(s). If the bank is online only and they have not added a beneficiary to their account, the next best thing is to download their statements. If they saved their statements on their computer or printed out hard copies every time the statements were available, this information eliminates the problem of their heirs accessing their accounts. Once they pass, their computer becomes part of their estate. The estate will then access the information on it, and they will then distribute that information according to the will. What the courts cannot do is access their online accounts through their computer.

What Happens to Music, E-Books and Photo-Sharing?

When they download a book onto their e-reader or a song from iTunes, they are granted a license to use the digital copy, but they do not own rights to it. If they are planning on sharing their curated iTunes collection, they better make sure they read the TOS to find out what they can or cannot pass on to their heirs.

The same goes with photo sharing. Everyone in the family might enjoy the memories of great vacations or the kid's or grandkid's graduation. If they use a photo sharing service like Flickr or Shutterfly so everyone in the family can enjoy the photos, and they want their heirs to have access to their digital photos after they are gone, they should save copies of all of their photos to their hard drive or a local back up — not the Cloud. This will make it much easier for cherished memories to stay in the family. It will also eliminate their heirs from having to go through thousands of digital images online after they pass.

Memories are the most important thing we leave behind. Make sure your loved one's memories are respected and protected.

Chapter 21: When Your Caregiving Responsibilities Are Over

The more you know, the better prepared you are to cope with the end-of-life responsibilities when your loved one passes.

In the chapter on emergency preparedness, we discussed creating a Survivor's Binder. It included a letter of instructions, funeral and/or burial arrangements, a will, and Digital Estates with a Master Password List. If your loved one created the letter of instruction and Master Password List, use these as a check list of whom to contact. This will help you at a time when your mind may be numb with shock and grief, and you are not certain what steps to take next.

It is important to note that joint accounts will be frozen at the time of your loved one's passing. If you do not have a separate checking, savings, or investment account in your name only, you will be unable to access your funds for daily living expenses or funerals or burial arrangements until the estate is settled through probate, which can take from a few months to a year or more. There are exceptions, consult a probate attorney for advice.

The following are the most common items you will need to deal with after your caregiving responsibilities are over.

Financial Responsibility

You are not responsible for your loved one's debt. There are a few exceptions. If you are a joint account holder on a bank account or credit card, you will be responsible for the account. If you co-signed on property with your loved one and your loved one was on Medicaid, the state may take action to recover the property and any other assets to cover the cost of care.

If you were taking care of a spouse, depending on your situation, you may have to pay for medical bills not covered by insurance or Medicare if applicable.

If your loved one went into a nursing home, did not have insurance, and was not covered by Medicaid, then you might be subject to Filial Support Laws. Filial Support Laws hold that the adult child of a parent with no means has the legal obligation to pay for the necessities of a parent who cannot pay for themselves, for example, nursing home care. In the states with Filial Support Laws on their books, the courts do not have to evenly divide up the obligations between the children but may choose the one who is most able to pay the debt. Nor do those states have to follow rulings from cases in other states. If Medicaid was in place, then the state will cover the cost of care.[85]

The Filial support laws have been on the books since before Medicare, Medicaid, and Social Security. After those measures were put in place as a safety net for seniors, the laws were no longer enforced. However, they weren't removed from their books, either. As the baby boomers age and require additional long-term care, the enforcement of these laws may increase as care providers try to recover their costs for elder care.

The following states and protectorate have some kind of filial support laws on their books as of 2019:

Alaska	Massachusetts	Puerto Rico
Arkansas	Mississippi	Rhode Island
California	Montana	South Dakota
Connecticut	Nevada	Tennessee
Delaware	New Jersey	Utah
Georgia	North Carolina	Vermont
Indiana	North Dakota	Virginia
Iowa	Ohio	West Virginia
Kentucky	Oregon	
Louisiana	Pennsylvania	

Contact an elder law attorney for advice on the best ways to help and protect your family. The National Academy of Elder Law Attorneys lists attorneys by state who are certified in elder law. Website: http://www.naela.org/.

Reporting to Social Security When a Family Member Dies

Social Security should be notified as soon as possible when a person dies. In most cases, the funeral director will report the person's death to Social Security. You will need to furnish the funeral director with the deceased's Social Security number so he or she can make the report. They will also be able to provide you with original issues of death certificates, usually for a minimal fee. You will need to know how many to purchase before you make funeral arrangements. See *How Many Death Certificates Do I Need?* Page 216.

Some of the deceased's family members may be able to receive Social Security benefits if the deceased person worked long enough under Social Security to qualify for benefits. You should get in touch with Social Security as soon as you can to make sure the family receives all of the benefits to which they may be entitled. Please read the following information carefully to learn what benefits may be available.

A one-time payment, called a death benefit, of $255 can be paid to the surviving spouse if he or she was living with the deceased; or, if living apart, was receiving certain Social Security benefits on the deceased's record. If there is no surviving spouse, the payment is made to a child who is eligible for benefits on the deceased's record in the month of death.

Certain family members may be eligible to receive monthly benefits, including:

- A widow or widower age 60 or older (age 50 or older if disabled)
- A surviving spouse at any age who is caring for the deceased's child under age 16 or disabled;
- an unmarried child of the deceased who is:
  - Younger than age 18 (or age 18 or 19 if he or she is a full-time student in an elementary or secondary school)
  - Age 18 or older with a disability that began before age 22
  - Age 62 or older, who were dependent on the deceased for at least half of their support
  - A surviving divorced spouse, under certain circumstances.

If the deceased was receiving Social Security benefits, you must return the benefit received for the month of death or subsequent months after death. For example, if the person dies in July, you must return the benefit paid in August. Keep in mind, the decedent must be alive for the entire month for the estate to keep the benefits.

Request through their bank that any funds received for the month of death or later be returned to Social Security. If the benefits were paid by check, do not cash any checks received for the month in which the person dies or later. Return the checks to Social Security as soon as possible.

To contact Social Security by phone: **1-800-772-1213.**

For more information you can go to their website: www.ssa.gov.

How Many Death Certificates Do I Need?

There are many organizations that require official death certificates as proof of a person's passing in order to close accounts, claim benefits, or settle estate claims. A legal aid can help you determine how many certificates you will need. However, there are several organizations that generally require an official death certificate.

Here is a list for your reference:

- Banks
  - Transfer individual checking or joint accounts

- o Transfer a savings account
- o Transfer certificates of deposit
- o Transfer a safe deposit box
- o Rolling over an IRA account
- Property: Mortgage companies and other property-related organizations
  - o Transfer each title of real estate
  - o Transfer ownership of a vehicle
- Government and Insurance
  - o Insurance claim including funeral home expenses
  - o Redeeming or transferring stocks, bonds, or treasury bills
  - o Federal and state tax returns
- Credit Bureaus
- Social Media Sites to complete Digital Estate activities

Some organizations will accept photocopies of the certificate. Having the right amount of death certificates will make this process less stressful during a time when you will be consumed by grief.

Credit Bureaus: Placing a Death Notice on Credit Reports

After a loved one dies, credit and finances are not going to be on the top of your mind. If you're handling the person's estate, it's important to know how to notify the credit bureaus and close his or her accounts.

According to Equifax.com, when someone passes away, his or her credit reports aren't closed automatically. However, once the four major credit bureaus – Equifax, Experian, Innovis, and TransUnion – are notified someone has died, their credit reports are sealed, and a death notice is placed on them.

This notification can happen in one of two ways: from the executor of the person's estate or from the Social Security Administration. Estate executors or court-appointed designees, however, are encouraged to contact each of the four major credit bureaus so the deceased's credit report will be flagged correctly.

Here are some steps you can take following the death of a loved one if you are the executor of the estate or court-appointed designee:

1. Contact the four major credit bureaus to find out what you need to do to notify them of someone's death and get a death notice placed on their credit reports.

A death notice flags a person's credit reports as "deceased - do not issue credit." If anyone tries to use the deceased person's information to apply for credit, the notice should be displayed telling the creditor the person is dead.

Determine what documents you will need to provide to the credit bureaus with for proof of the person's death, along with proof that you are the authorized designee. The required documents may vary, based on your relationship with the deceased—whether he or she is a parent or spouse, for instance—and based on each credit bureau's requirement.

The required information might include:

- The person's legal name
- The person's Social Security number
- The person's date of birth and date of death
- A copy of the death certificate
- Copies of any required legal documents
- Your full name
- Your address (to send confirmation of death notice placement)

If you are also requesting a copy of the person's credit report, you will need a copy of a government-issued ID, such as a driver's license or passport.

2. Mail the required documents to the credit bureaus. Make copies of everything you send. Send the documents via certified mail.

3. Review the deceased person's credit reports to understand what open accounts they have with creditors and lenders. It's a good idea to request copies of credit reports from each of the four major credit bureaus, since not all lenders and creditors report to all four.

You may need to contact lenders and creditors to notify them the person is deceased, and the accounts need to be closed, even if the account has a zero balance. Lender and creditor contact information can be found on the credit reports. You may be required to provide a copy of the person's death certificate and other legal documents. A joint account may remain open even after one of the people has died.

How do I obtain a deceased person's credit report?

The spouse or executor of the estate may request the deceased person's credit report by mailing a request to each of the credit bureaus.

Send a letter along with the following information about the deceased:

- Legal name
- Social Security Number
- Date of birth
- Date of death
- Last known address
- A copy of the death certificate or letters testamentary.

Also send information about yourself, including:

- Your full name

> A *letters testamentary*, also known as letters of testamentary, is a document issued by a court or public official authorizing the executor of a will to take control of a deceased person's estate.

- Address for sending final confirmation
- In the case of an executor, include the court order or other document showing that you are an executor.

Send the request and information to all four credit reporting companies by mail:

Equifax P.O. Box 105139 Atlanta, GA 30348-5139	TransUnion P.O. Box 2000 Chester, PA 19016
Experian P.O. Box 2002 Allen, TX 75013	Innovis PO Box 1689 Pittsburgh, PA 15230-1689

It is important to get the death notice placed within two weeks of a person's death.

If you receive calls from debt collectors after someone's death, you do not have to speak with them about the debts of a deceased relative—unless you are a joint account holder. *If you are not a joint account holder do not give out any personal information.*

Report any problems with a debt collector to your State Attorney General's Office.

Unclaimed Money and Property

The last item you will want to take care of, if you have not already done so, is search for any monies owed to your loved one. Start your search using the U.S. government's website www.usa.gov/unclaimed-money. It gives advice on where to start searching for any monies and property owed to your loved one's estate.

You should never receive a phone call from someone claiming to be from the government who offers to send you unclaimed property for a fee. Government agencies will not call you about unclaimed money or property.[86]

Disposal of Unused Medications

When your loved one passes, there may be unused prescription medications that will need to be disposed of. At the time of this writing, the following nationwide pharmacies have programs to take back unused over the counter and prescription medications:

- CVS Pharmacy
- Rite Aid
- Walgreens

Walgreens will accept unused prescription, no matter which pharmacy dispensed them. Check with your local pharmacy to see if they have a medication take-back program. None of the programs accept illegal drugs, used needles, or paraphernalia.

With the growing opioid epidemic, many pharmacies offer DisposeRX packets to customers with opioid prescriptions. The packets include a powder, that can be poured into the prescription bottles. When combined with water, it creates a gel around the medication that can be discarded with household trash or taken to a drug-collection location.[87]

If you are having difficulties finding a place to dispose of unused medications, the National Association of Boards of Pharmacy offers on their website a national drug disposal locator: https://nabp.pharmacy/initiatives/awarxe/drug-disposal-locator/

Twice a year the Drug Enforcement Agency (DEA) collects expired or unused prescription medications through its National Prescription Drug Take Back Days in April and October.

If you do not have any of these options available, then you can mix the unused medications (do not crush any tablets or capsules) with dirt, kitty litter, or used coffee grounds. Place them in a sealable, airtight plastic bag, and disposed of them with your household trash.

Chapter 22: We've Come to the End of this Journey

"You cannot teach a man anything, only help him to find it within himself." ~Galileo

When my husband and I started the caregiving journey with my family, we had no idea what we were doing. The saying, "You don't know, what you don't know, until you know it," comes to mind. Like many before us, we staggered blindly through the dark maze of caregiving, searching for answers, including to my father's question, "I have Alzheimer's, not the plague. What will it take to be treated like a human being?"

Which led us here to the end of this book. We've covered a lot of material. Use what works for you. Don't try to do everything. Pick a chapter and work through it. Make mistakes, forgive yourself, and try again. Dementia will wipe the slate clean for you, sometimes in ten minutes. Your loved one won't remember the mistakes, only the feelings.

Dementia caregiving is hard.

Make time to take care of yourself. Make time to breathe deeply. Make time to slow down and enjoy the small moments. Remember the importance of touch and expressing your love and your receiving it in return. Share with your family and friends how to visit and help. Accept the help that is offered to you. Allow yourself to have fun.

Make time to laugh.

When it's all over, what's really important are the good memories that remain. The funny mistakes, the oops. Laughing so hard you snorted a beverage out your nose. Give yourself time to heal.

The good memories stay and, in time, the bad ones drift away.

When my father disappeared through the smog-filled tunnel of dementia, he no longer remembered his sister, my sisters, my husband, or me. While he could still speak, he would repeat his favorite stanza of a counting rhyme.

"Wire, briar, limber lock,
Three geese in a flock,
One flew east, one flew west,
One flew over the cuckoo's nest."
A fitting rhyme for someone with Alzheimer's Disease.

When my father died, his not remembering me faded. What remained: blowing bubbles in our milkshakes, fishing on the open ocean and puking up our lunches, his saying, "I've got big hands"—and reciting nursery rhymes.

At the end of your caregiving journey, what will you remember? Will you remember the things that made you laugh? Will you remember the things that made you cry? Will you remember the ones you love? Will you look back with regret, with pride, with joy?

What will you find within yourself?

May you always remember the funny moments, the shared laugh, a moment of connection. May you send your guilt on that first class, one-way ticket to the Bermuda Triangle—you've already funded the fare in full. And as you go forth, may you help others on their journey find their way back to healing too.

* * *

"It's bad to suppress laughter. It goes back down and spreads to your hips." ~Fred Allen

Now go have a tee hee moment, you've earned it.

APPENDICES

Appendix A

This is for example purposes only. Your needs and directions will be different. This does not take the place of medical advice.

Example Medication List

Medication lists are useful for doctor's appoints, hospital admissions, and any time emergency medical technicians (EMTs) are called upon.

Include the patient's full name and date of birth (DOB) and the name of her primary care physician (PCP) at the top of the form. In addition to all prescriptions, include all over-the-counter medications and supplements. Supplements can cause adverse drug interactions. Include two more columns: (1) Column for the date the medication was started. This will help you identify if a sudden behavior change might be caused by a new drug interaction. (2) Column for whether the medication is taken with or without food.

Name: Myrna Vander Beek　　　**DOB: 11/27/45**　　**PCP: Collin Uphill, MD. Updated: 11/17/20**

Medication & Strength	Dose	Directions	Reason for Medication	Administration Time	Prescribing Doctor
Lantus	25 units a.m. / 35 units p.m.	Shot with needle twice daily	Long-acting Insulin	7:30 a.m. and 6:00 p.m.	Trenton
Galantamine	4 mg	Orally, Twice Daily	Alzheimer/Dementia	7:30 a.m. and 6:00 p.m.	Uphill
Aspirin	81 mg	Orally, Once Daily	Modest Pain and Heart	8:00 a.m.	Uphill

Sometimes your loved one may have allergic reactions to medications. Include a list of known medication allergies:

Medication Allergies	Symptom
Aricept	Stops eating
Seraquel	Blood sugar levels over 350 mg/dl and uncontrolled eating.
Lorazapam	Hyperactivity
Plavix	Excessive stomach bleeding, body pain, lethargy

Example Appointment Schedule

With aging comes increased risks for chronic illnesses outside of dementia. Keeping track of doctor's appointments, specialists, and where they are located can become a chore when you are trying to balance the rest of your life too. Keeping track of appointments, plus upcoming medical procedures can prevent missed appointments or double-booking appointments.

Here is a sample sheet for your reference:

Date	Time	Doctor	Comments
April 11	4:00 PM	Dr. Bones	Knee evaluation.
April 30	1:30 PM	Dr. Backer	Kidney follow-up
May 8	2:45 PM	Dr. Hart	Cardiac follow-up, annual exam
May 9	1:00 PM	Cardiac Study Center	Dial-up pacemaker check
May 9	2:00 PM	Dr. Bones	Pre-surgery knee evaluation.
May 9	3:30 PM	Pre-Admit Clinic-General Hosp.	Blood work prior to surgery
May 15	7:30 AM	Dr. Bones	Right knee surgery
May 30	3:20 PM	Dr. Bones	Post-surgery knee evaluation and staple removal.

Pending	Comments
August 12	Hip Surgery pending blood sugar results by Dr. Trenton
September 13	Left knee Surgery pending evaluation by Dr. Bones

Addresses

Dr. Uphill/Dr. Backer
1901 Whoop-it-Up Way, Ste C201 (Anytown)

Health Insurance
Medicare Plans A and B
Coverage Number: 1WE4RP0LY35T3R

Cardiac Center/Dr. Hart
1901 Whoop-it-Up Way, Ste C301 (Anytown)

Doctor	Specialty	Phone	Fax
Dr. Collin Uphill	PCP	555-792-MAIN	555-792-COPY
Dr. Dem Bones	Hip Doctor	555-301-HIPS	555-761-KNEE
General Hospital-Jill Pill	Social Svcs	555-459-SVCS	
Dr. G.F.R. Backer	Kidney Doctor	555-5KI-DNEY	555-30S-TONE
Cardiac Center: Dr. Gotta Hart	Pace Maker	555-57H-EART	555-574-TAVR
—Lilly, Device Appt. Scheduler	Pace Maker	555-396-PACE	
Dr. Lada Trenton	Diabetes	55D-IAB-ETES	555-INS-ULIN
Dr. Fun Gus Eddy	Foot Doctor	55A-THL-ETES	555-623-FOOT

Dr. Bones
1550 Medical Blvd, #210 (Anytown)

Dr. Trenton
1710 Medical Blvd, #110 (Anytown)

Dr. Eddy
1901 Whoop-it-Up Way, Ste C205 (Anytown)

At the time of this writing, medical practitioners still use fax machines. Knowing fax numbers for each of your medical practitioners' offices cans speed up communication between offices and labs when you are scheduling medical procedures if they are not within the same network.

212

Appendix B

Preparing Your Living Environment

<u>Items that make life easier for older adults with mild cognitive impairment:</u>

- Recliners
- Heating pads with auto shut off
- Special cushions for thin people or people with sensitive skin
- Clip-on lighting that attaches to shelves or cabinets for areas that need more lighting
- Magnifying glasses
- Reaching tools for items dropped on the floor or on a high shelf
  - 32" Grabber-Reacher
  - 19" Grabber-Reacher
- Socks Aid (for putting on socks)
- 28" Dressing Aid Stick (for putting on shirts, pulling up pants, removing socks)
- 24" long shoehorn
- Jar opening devices includes automatic jar opener
- Foam tubing can be used to make almost any type of utensil or tool easier to grip
- Writing grips for pens and pencils
- Adaptive foam or rubber handles
- Universal knob turner can be used with the bathtub, stove top, microwave, dishwasher or washing machine (useful for people with arthritis)
- Key holder designed for arthritis patients are brightly colored and can help in the search for lost keys
- Steps for getting into the bathtub
- Inflatable bath pillows to aid in reclining comfortably in the bathtub
- Long-handled back brush or sponge for bathing
- Toilet safety frame
- A bidet for cleaning their private parts
- Toilet bidet (attaches to existing toilet, does not require additional bathroom space)
- Handheld showerhead

<u>Items for adults with moderate cognitive impairment:</u>

- Shower chair
- Cane
- Walker
- Wheelchair
- Blood pressure cuff
- Digital thermometer
- Mediscope (used for checking eyes, ears and throat for signs of infection)
- First aid supplies
- Pill minders
- Incontinence supplies
- Sitz bath
- Sponge-tipped swabs with toothpaste
- Floss picks
- Nonslip bathtub mats or nonslip stickers or decals
- Dycem nonslip material
- Grab bars
- Raised toilet seat
- Padded toilet seat for people who have soft skin or have to sit for long periods of time
- Portable commode
- Commode liners
- Urinal or bed pan
- Baby bumpers for table corners
- No-tie shoelaces
- Dimmer switches to raise lighting levels as the sun goes down
- Battery operated door alarms
- Radiant wall heater for the bathroom
- Swivel cushion for the car for people who have mobility issues, it raises the seat slightly and makes it easier to get into and out of a car
- Car Caddie, a nylon strap attached to the car door window frame, when fitted appropriately, acts as a sturdy place to hold onto when exiting the car
- Adaptive car door handles also known as "handibars" for car door support can help with stability getting into and out of a car. They latch to the car door on both the driver and passenger doors

Appendix C

The Meltdown Trigger List

Here is a blank Meltdown Trigger List:

Look for the common activity in each event	Event 1	Event 2	Event 3
Date, Day, Time			
Location			
Descriptions of physical surrounding with activities			
Identify common event(s)			
Distraction techniques that work			

If you would like to download a free template for the Meltdown Trigger List, go to my website: tracycramperkins.com/resources. Select *Useful Forms* from the menu.

Resources

Because caregiving is so stress-filled, you need all the help you can get. Whether you are new to caregiving or have been caring for someone with dementia for years, here are some resources which might help you. Websites and blogs change or disappear regularly. If the link to one of these resources is broken, check my website www.tracycramperkins.com/resources for updates. If you don't see an update let me know through my contact page.

Useful Websites

Advanced Directives

AARP Advanced Directive Forms: https://www.aarp.org/caregiving/financial-legal/free-printable-advance-directives/. They are free, state-specific advanced directive forms and instructions.

Health Care Directive for Dementia: www.dementia-directive.org

Area Agencies on Aging (AAA)

Association of Area Agencies on Aging: www.n4a.org

Adaptive Clothing

Silverts: www.silverts.com
Buck and Buck: www.buckandbuck.com
Dignity Resource Council: www.dignityrc.org. Modesty garments for bathing and toileting.

Assisted Living

Argentum: www.argentum.org. They provide information and resources on assisted living option and how to locate them.

Credit Monitoring Services

Equifax: www.equifax.com or by phone: 1-866-349-5191
Experian: www.experian.com or by phone: 1-800-493-1058
Innovis: www.innovis.com or by phone: 1-800-540-2505
TransUnion: www.transunion.com or by phone: 1-800-916-8800
Annual Free Credit Report: www.annualcreditreport.com

Deafness and Dementia

Alzheimer's Scotland offers information designed specifically for caregivers of members of the Deaf community, those with acquired hearing loss, those who are deaf and blind and those working with additional physical disabilities. They provide a PDF format caregiver guide in English. Website: https://www.alzscot.org/our-work/dementia-support/information-sheets/dementia-and-deafness

Driving

American Occupational Therapy Association's: https://myaota.aota.org/driver_search/index.aspx

Automobile Association of America's Helping Seniors Drive Safer and Longer Program which includes professional driving assessments. For more information visit: https://seniordriving.aaa.com/evaluate-your-driving-ability/professional-assessment/

AARP Driver Safety Course: https://www.aarpdriversafety.org/

Distraction Technique Aids

Joy for All Companion Pets from Ageless Innovations, website: **joyforall.com** or by phone: 866-532-8531. They offer robotic cats, kittens, and puppies for those suffering from loneliness and dementia. Those with dementia may not understand the robots are not real and the "animals" make great substitute pets and creates a sense of calm and promotes happiness and play.

Do No Call Registry

National Do Not Call Registry: www.donotcall.gov

Document Preparation and Organization

AARP's *Prepare to Care* **guide**, there is an in-depth section at the end of the guide which includes a place to list your loved one's legal, financial and medical contacts with spaces for medications, their Medicare information, VA Benefits, which bills are due and when, passwords and a host of other things you will need to know to prepare for that next step. Visit: https://www.aarp.org/content/dam/aarp/home-and-family/caregiving/2012-10/PrepareToCare-Guide-FINAL.pdf

Elder Abuse

National Center on Elder Abuse Hotline: https://ncea.acl.gov/Resources/State.aspx

National Adult Protective Services Association: http://www.napsa-now.org/get-help/help-in-your-area/

National Council on Child Abuse & Family Violence: https://www.preventfamilyviolence.org/adult-protective-services-numbers

National Domestic Violence Hotline: www.thehotline.org or by phone 800-799-7233

National Long-Term Care Ombudsman Resource Center: http://theconsumervoice.org/get_help For use in nursing home or adult family homes.

Elder Law

Lists attorneys who are certified in elder law by state:

The National Academy of Elder Law Attorneys: https://www.naela.org/.

The National Elder Law Foundation: https://nelf.org/search/custom.asp?id=5427

Emergency Preparedness

American Red Cross: www.redcross.org

Center for Disease Control (CDC): emergency.cdc.gov

Federal Emergency Management Agency (FEMA) main website: www.fema.gov

Federal Emergency Management Agency (FEMA) Emergency Preparedness: www.ready.gov

Grab and Go Backpack: www.mil.wa.gov/preparedness

Take Winter by Storm: takewinterbystorm.org (This website was created for Washington State, however, the information works for any weather related disaster.)

End of Life Care

Get Palliative Care: www.getpalliativecare.org/provider-directory. This site is run by the Center to Advance Palliative Care, a national organization dedicated to increasing the availability of palliative care services. They provide a listing by state.

Medicare: www.medicare.gov/hospicecompare. Medicare provides ratings for hospice agencies.

> Medicare.gov created a new website for comparing all provider types. Visit it at www.medicare.gov/care-compare

National Association for Home Care & Hospice: www.nahc.org. Consumer information on how to select a home care provider or hospice provider.

National Association of Social Workers: www.socialworkers.org. They also have a directory of licensed social workers at www.helppro.com/nasw.

National Hospice and Palliative Care Organization: www.nhpco.org or 800-646-6460

The Conversation Project: www.theconversationproject.org. This group was created to help people talk about their end-of-life care wishes.

Financial Management

American Association of Daily Money Managers to monitor bank accounts and credit cards: secure.aadmm.com

Group Caregiving

ShareTheCare, Inc.: www.sharethecare.org. This organization provides support and guidance for group caregiving to those who are seriously ill, disabled, or have dementia.

Village to Village Network: www.vtvnetwork.org. They are an organization who helps communities start Villages. Villages are membership-based groups who respond to the needs of older people within a geographic area.

Health Care Directive for Dementia

Dementia Directive: www.dementia-directive.org

Health Insurance and Medication

Centers for Medicare & Medicaid Services: www.cms.gov. This website provides information connecting you to Medicare, Medicaid, and the Health Insurance Exchanges.

Medlineplus: www.medlineplus.gov. This site is run by the National Institutes of Health and the United States National Library of Medicine. The website has information on over 600 health topics including the current information on A.D. and dementia. It also includes information on prescription and over-the-counter drugs and a medical encyclopedia.

The National Council on Aging: www.benefitscheckup.org. This website helps people age 55 and older locate programs that may pay for a portion or all of their prescription drug costs, healthcare, utilities, and other services. Fill out the questionnaire and the site will direct you to programs in your area.

Needymeds: www.needymeds.org or by phone 800-503-6897. Needymeds finds help with the cost of medications.

State Health Insurance Assistance Program (SHIP): www.shiptacenter.org or by phone 877-839-2675. SHIP offers one-on-one counselling for people with Medicare and their families.

State Pharmaceutical Assistance Program:
https://www.medicare.gov/pharmaceutical-assistance-program/state-programs.aspx.

Medicaid: www.medicaid.gov. Each state has its own Medicaid program. Go to the *Resources for States* to be directed to the Medicaid website for your area.

Home Modifications

American Academy of Healthcare Interior Designers (AAHID): www.aahid.org

National Association of Home Builders:
www.nahb.org/NAHB-Community/Directories. Choose "Professionals with Home Building Designations" and choose the filter for "CAPS." It is the online directory of certified aging-in-place specialists who can do home modifications that make a home more accessible and safer.

ADABathroom.com: http://www.adabathroom.com/index

Canva: https://www.canva.com/colors/combinations/ Their color design wiki gives information about different color combinations when choosing contrasting colors to help your loved one navigate their living space longer.

Incontinence Pads

Pooch pads: www.poochpad.com. They carry machine washable pads with odor control built in.

Locating Adult Day Care or In-home Care

A Place for Mom: www.aplaceformom.com
Eldercare Locator: www.eldercare.acl.gov or by phone 800 677-1116
National Adult Day Services Association: www.nadsa.org
Home Instead: www.homeinstead.com or by phone 888-331-1023 (U.S. only), Rest of the World 1-402-205-8392
Visiting Angels: www.visitingangelsseniorcare.com

Long-Term Care Facilities

American Elder Care Research Organization: www.payingforseniorcare.com or by phone: 641-715-3900 ext. 606151#. This website helps people find ways to pay for eldercare.

Continuing Care Accreditation Commission: www.carf.org This organizations monitors continuing care retirement communities.

Genworth Cost of Care Calculator:
www.genworth.com/aging-and-you/finances/cost-of-care.html

This website calculates and compares the cost of care for in-home care, community and assisted living and nursing home facilities.

LeadingAge: www.leadingage.org. They provide consumer information on long-term care facilities and services, and the best ways to access them.

National Clearinghouse for Long-Term Care Information: http://www.longtermcare.gov/. This site provides information and tools for selecting long-term care.

Medicare's Nursing Home Compare: http://www.medicare.gov/nursinghomecompare/search.html or by phone 800-633-4227.

Medicare.gov created a new website for comparing all provider types. Visit it at www.medicare.gov/care-compare

Meal Services

Meals on Wheels Association of America: www.mealsonwheelsamerica.org or by phone 703-548-5558

Medical Documents

National POLST Paradigm: www.polst.org

Medication Disposal Services

National Association of Boards of Pharmacy, Drug Disposal Locator: https://nabp.pharmacy/initiatives/awarxe/drug-disposal-locator/
U.S. Drug Enforcement Agency (DEA) National Drug Take Back Days: https://takebackday.dea.gov/
Walgreen Medication Disposal Locations finder: https://www.walgreens.com/storelocator/find.jsp?RxDisposal=true

Military Support Services

Elizabeth Dole Foundations: www.elizabethdolefoundation.org

Veterans Affairs: www.caregiver.va.gov or by phone 855-260-3274. They provide support and services for families caring for veterans. They connect caregivers with local support programs.

We Honor Veterans: www.wehonorveterans.org is a program of the National Hospice and Palliative Care Organization. They help hospice and community organizations meet the unique needs of America's Veterans and their families.

Memory Kits

WebJunction: https://www.webjunction.org/news/webjunction/memory-kits.html. Library Based Memory Kits, from activities to famous photos and informational booklets were created for this project with dementia and Alzheimer's Disease to help remember moments from their past. Check with your local library.

Positive Approaches to Caregiving

Jolene Brackey: https://www.enhancedmoments.com/. She offers training videos and classes for dementia care using her enhanced moments method.

Teepa Snow: www.teepasnow.com She offers training videos and classes for dementia care using her positive approach method.

Respite Organizations

ARCH National Respite Network: www.archrespite.org. It is an organization that helps locate respite services.

Support Services

AARP Local Caregiver Resources Guide: www.aarp.org/caregiverresourceguides

AARP Prepare to Care Guide: https://www.aarp.org/content/dam/aarp/home-and-family/caregiving/2012-10/PrepareToCare-Guide-FINAL.pdf

Administrations on Community Living (ACL): www.acl.gov. It is the federal agency responsible for advancing the interests of older people. There are an assortment of tools and information for older adults and family caregivers.

African Americans Against Alzheimer's:
www.usagainstalzheimers.org/networks/african-americans It is an organization dedicated to address and eliminate Alzheimer's Disease, including among African Americans.

African American Alzheimer's & Wellness Association:
https://www.africanamericanalz.org/ or by phone 800-489-6040. It is an organization that supports aging African Americans.

Alzheimer's Association: www.alz.org or by phone 800-272-3900

Alzheimer's Association Driving Contract: www.alz.org/driving

ALZ Connected is the Alzheimer's Associations online community forum: www.alzconnected.org. This forum is for anyone who is affected by A.D. and other dementias.

Alzheimer's Caregiver Support Online: www.alzonline.net. This site is sponsored by the University of Florida. It offers useful information for caregivers.

Alzheimer's Foundation of America: www.alzfdn.org. They are committed to improving the quality of life for A.D. patients and their families.

Care.com: www.care.com. They have services to connect families with caregivers.

Caregiver Action Network: www.caregiveraction.org or by phone 202-454-3970. They provide information and support for the family caregivers.

Careinginfo: www.caringinfo.org. They provide support for end-of-life care through the national Hospice and Palliative Care Organization: www.nhpco.org/patients-and-caregivers

Daily Caring: www.dailycaring.com. They provide information covering daily care, caregiver stress, senior health, senior housing, finances and legal advice.

Dementia Society of America: dementiasociety.org or by phone 800-DEMENTIA (800-336-3684). They are an all-volunteer organization that provides information, resources, and a web-based locator to help caregivers find local support.

Death with Dignity: www.deathwithdignity.org

Family Caregiver Alliance: www.caregiver.org or by phone 800-445-8106

Leeza's Care Connection: www.leezascareconnection.org. The Leeza Gibbons Memory Foundation offers resources for caregivers including information about A.D., caregiving, legal, and financial matters.

National Alliance for Caregiving: www.caregiving.org. They provide support for improving the quality of life for caregivers and those they care for.

National Alliance for Hispanic Health: www.healthyamericas.org. They have the Hispanic Family Health Helpline at 866-783-2645 which supplies free and confidential health information for Hispanic families.

National Association for Home Care & Hospice: www.nahc.org. Consumer information on how to select a home care provider or hospice provider.

National Association of Social Workers: www.socialworkers.org. They also have a directory of licensed social workers at www.helppro.com/nasw.

National Institute on Aging Alzheimer's Disease and Related Dementias: www.nia.nih.gov/health/alzheimers or by phone 800-438-4380

National Poison Control Center: www.poison.org or 1-800-222-1222

National Suicide Prevention Lifeline: www.suicidepreventionlifeline.org or 1-800-273-8255

Psychology Today: https://www.psychologytoday.com/us/therapists/grief for mental health professionals listed by state.

SAGEUSA: www.sageusa.org/resource-category/caregiving/. An organization who provides counseling, information, support groups to gay, lesbian, bisexual and transgender caregivers.

Social Security Administration: www.ssa.gov or by phone 800-772-1213

Well Spouse Association: www.wellspouse.org. They are a non-profit and have local chapters around the country who offer face-to-face and telephone support groups for spouses.

The Women's Alzheimer's Movement: www.thewomensalzheimersmovement.org. Founded by Maria Shriver, it covers brain health advice and stories for caregivers along with other resources.

2-1-1: www.211.org. This is a free and confidential service for people across North America to find the local resources they need.

U.S. Department of Health & Human Services: hhs.gov/aging/state-resources. List available programs and services by state.

United States Postal Service Informed Delivery:
https://informeddelivery.usps.com/box/pages/intro/start.action This free services allows you to see what is arriving in the mail each day to monitor for fraudulent activities.

Vaccine Finder: vaccinefinder.org/find-vaccine This free service from the Centers for Disease Control and Prevention (CDC) that helps you locate vaccine supplies, such as flu vaccines, in your area by zip code.

<u>Translation Languages</u>

Alzheimer's Association (U.S.): http://www.alz.org/alzheimers_disease_4719.asp
The Alzheimer's Association provides an interactive tour of the brain in multiple languages. Go to bottom of the website's page and select a language.

Languages: Arabic, Chinese, Finnish, French, German, Hindi, Italian, Japanese, Korean, Polish, Portuguese, Russian, Spanish, Vietnamese.

Alzheimer's Association (U.S.) Spanish Portal: https://alz.org/ayuda-y-apoyo?_ga=2.1104820.46702545.1584470603-144415759.1580964892

The Alzheimer's Association's Spanish Portal offers a variety of articles in Spanish.

Languages: Spanish

Family Caregiver Alliance (U.S.): https://www.caregiver.org/other-languages

The Family Caregiver Alliance provides a guide to Early-Stage Alzheimer's.

Languages: English, Spanish, Chinese, Korean, Vietnamese.

Alzheimer's Society U.K.: https://www.alzheimers.org.uk/publications-about-dementia/the-dementia-guide-other-languages

The Alzheimer's Society U.K. provides a list of factsheets and booklets.

Languages: Bengali, Gujarati, Hindi, Punjabi, Traditional Chinese, Urdu, Welsh

Alzheimer's Scotland:

https://www.alzscot.org/our-work/dementia-support/information-sheets/dementia-and-deafness

The provide dementia resources for the Deaf Community.

Languages: English

DeafDOC.ORG: deafdoc.org.

It provides health education for the Deaf and Hard of Hearing Community, Interpreters, and Healthcare professionals.

Languages: English and American Sign Language (ASL)

Dementia Australia: https://www.dementia.org.au/languages

Dementia Australia provides dementia resources in many languages.

Languages: Arabic, Armenian, Assyrian, Chinese, Croatian, Dari, Dutch, Finnish, French, German, Greek, Hindi, Hungarian, Indonesian, Italian, Japanese, Khmer, Korean, Laotian, Latvian, Lithuanian, Macedonian, Maltese, Nepali, Polish, Portuguese, Punjabi, Romanian, Russian, Serbian, Spanish, Tagalog, Tamil, Thai, Turkish, Ukrainian, Vietnamese.

Latino Alzheimer's and Memory Disorders Alliance:

http://www.latinoalzheimersalliance.org/

The Latino Alzheimer's and Memory Disorders Alliance provides education and support programs in the Latino communities of Illinois and creates awareness.

Languages: English, Spanish

Agency for Healthcare Research and Quality: http://www.ahrq.gov/health-care-information/informacion-en-espanol/index.html

The Agency for Healthcare Research and Quality's Spanish language resources provide translated guides on many topics.

Language: Spanish

FamilyDoctor.org: http://familydoctor.org/familydoctor/es.html

FamilyDoctor.org provides family doctor pamphlets in Spanish.

Language: Spanish

Healthfinder: http://www.healthfinder.gov/espanol/

Part of the U.S. Department of Health and Human Services, Healthfinder offers translated Spanish language resources on various conditions.

Language: Spanish

The National Network of Libraries of Medicine: *https://nnlm.gov/consumer-health-information-many-languages-resources*

Multilingual Health Information (encompasses all health issues, not just dementia).

Languages: Arabic, Cambodian/Khmer, Chinese, French, German, Hmong, Korean, Laotian, Russian, Spanish, Thai, Vietnamese.

Health Information Translations: https://www.healthinfotranslations.org/

Health Information Translations provides health resources and information for health care professionals and others seeking material in communities with limited understanding of English. This website is provided by the Ohio State University Wexner Medical Center, Mount Carmel Health System, Ohio Health and Nationwide Children's Hospital.

Languages: Amharic, Arabic, Bosnian, Chinese Simplified, Chinese Traditional, English, French, Hindi, Japanese, Khmer, Korean, Marshallese, Nepali, Portuguese, Russian, Somali, Spanish, Swahili, Tagalog, Tigrinya, Ukrainian, Vietnamese.

Health Translations Online Directory (Australia):
http://www.healthtranslations.vic.gov.au/

The Health Translations Online Directory allows health care professionals and others working in diverse communities to find easily accessible translated health information. Based in Victoria, Australia, the directory provides links to information from Victoria, Australia, in addition to other countries and regions.

Languages: Afrikaans, Akan, Albanian, Amharic, Arabic, Armenian, Assyrian, Auslan, Bemba, Bengali, Bosnian, Bulgarian, Burmese, Chaldean, Chin, Chin Hakha, Chinese Simplified, Chinese Traditional, Croatian, Czech, Danish, Dari, Dinka, Dutch, English, Estonian, Faili, Farsi (Persian), Fijian, Finnish, French, German, Greek, Gujarati, Hakka, Hazaragi, Hebrew, Hindi, Hmong, Hungarian, Igbon, Indonesian, Italian, Japanese, Juba Arabic, Karen, Khmer (Cambodian), Kirundi, Korean, Krio, Kurdish, Kurmanji, Lao, Latvian, Lebanese Arabic, Lingala, Lithuanian, Macedonian, Malay, Malayalam, Maltese, Maori, Maori (Cook Islands) Mizo, Nepali, Norwegian, Nuer, Oromo, Pashto, Polish, Portuguese, Punjabi, Romanian, Russian, Samoan, Serbian, Serbian (Cyrillic), Serbian (Latin), Sinhalese, Slovak, Slovene, Somali, Sorani, Spanish, Sudanese, Sudanese Arabic, Swahili, Swahili (Congolese), Swahili (Kenyan), Swedish, Tagalog, Tamil, Telugu, Tetum, Thai, Tibetan, Tigrinya, Tok Pisin, Tongan, Turkish, Ukrainian, Urdu, Vietnamese, Yiddish, Zomi.

Lab Tests Online: https://labtestsonline.org/global-sites

Lab Tests Online provides peer-reviewed articles in plain language to help patients understand their lab tests so they can understand and discuss them more easily with their physicians.

Languages: English, Spanish, Italian, French, Greek, Turkish, Czech, Hungarian, Polish, Portuguese, Chinese, Korean.

National Library of Medicine:

http://www.nlm.nih.gov/medlineplus/languages/languages.html

Information for patients and health care professionals from the National Library of Medicine's consumer health website Medlineplus.

Languages: Arabic, Amharic, Bengali, Bosnian, Burmese, Chamorro, Chinese Simplified, Chinese Traditional, Chuukese, Croatian, Farsi, French, German, Gujarathi, Haitian Creole, Hindi, Hmong, Ilocano, Italian, Japanese, Karen, Khmer, Kirundi, Korean, Kurdish, Laotian, Marshallese, Nepali, Oromo, Polish, Portuguese, Punjabi, Romanian, Russian, Samoan, Somali, Spanish, Swahili, Tagalog, Thai, Tigrinya, Tongan, Turkish, Ukrainian, Urdu, Vietnamese, and more.

HealthReach, Health Information in Many Languages:

https://healthreach.nlm.nih.gov/#

HealthReach is a database that provides multilingual, multicultural health information and patient education materials about both health conditions and wellness topics.

Languages: Albanian, Amharic, Arabic, Armenian, Bengali, Bosnian, Burmese, Cape Verdean Creole, Chinese Simplified, Chinese Traditional, Chuukese, Dzongkha (Bhutanese), English, Farsi, French, German, Gujarati, Haitian Creole, Hakha Chin, Hindi, Hmong, Ilocano, Indonesian, Italian, Japanese, Karen, Karenni, Khmer, Kinyarwanda, Kirundi, Korean, Kurdish, Lao, Levantine (Arabic dialect), Malay, Marshallese, Modern Standard Arabic, Nepali, Oromo, Pashto, Pohnpeian, Polish, Portuguese, Punjabi, Russian, Samoan, Serbo-Croatian, Somali, Spanish, Sudanese (Arabic dialect), Swahili, Tagalog, Thai, Tibetan, Tigrinya, Tongan, Turkish, Ukrainian, Urdu, Vietnamese, Yiddish.

SAGEUSA: www.sageusa.org.

An organization who provides counseling, information, support groups to gay, lesbian, bisexual, and transgender caregivers.

Languages: English and Spanish

University of Washington, Harborview Medical Center Ethnomed: https://ethnomed.org/about/interpreter-services/.

They use interpreters skilled in speaking in over 80 different dialects and languages when someone has been hospitalized.

Unclaimed Money or Property

The United States Government: www.usa.gov/unclaimed-money. This website has links to all 50 state so you can search for unclaimed money or property.

Wandering

MedicAlert Foundation and the Alzheimer's Association:
www.medicalert.org/alzheimers-dementia Phone 1-800-432-5378 or to donate to the Alzheimer's Association, 30 percent of a new membership (no additional cost to you) is donated via this link: https://www.medicalert.org/alz

Alzheimer's Association Safe Return:
www.alz.org/help-support/caregiving/safety/medicalert-with-24-7-wandering-support this site ensures automatic donation. This is the same program as above but through the Alzheimer's Association website portal.

SafetyNet Tracking Systems by LoJack: safetynettracking.com/ or phone 1-877-434-6384 Uses RFID or GPS

Notes

1. Cousins, Norman, *Anatomy of an Illness as Perceived by the Patient*, New York, W.W. Norton & Company, 1979, 2001, 2005.

2. Goodheart, Annette, *Laughter Therapy, How to Laugh About Everything in Your Life That Isn't Really Funny*, Santa Barbara, Less Stress Press, 1994. Pages 17-19.

3. Gerloff, Pamela, "You're Not Laughing Enough, and That's No Joke," Psychology Today, June 21, 2011.
   https://www.psychologytoday.com/us/blog/the-possibility-paradigm/201106/youre-not-laughing-enough-and-thats-no-joke

4. Scott, Paula Spencer, *Surviving Alzheimer's, Practical Tips and Soul-Saving Wisdom for Caregivers*, Second Edition, San Francisco, Eva Birch Media, 2018. Page 23.

5. Gerloff, Pamela, "You're Not Laughing Enough, and That's No Joke," Psychology Today, June 21, 2011
   https://www.psychologytoday.com/us/blog/the-possibility-paradigm/201106/youre-not-laughing-enough-and-thats-no-joke.

6. Chapman, Daniel P., PhD, MSc, Sheree Marshall Williams, PhD, MSc, Tara W. Strine, MPH, Robert F. Anda, MD, MS, Margaret J. Moore, MPH, "Dementia and Its Implications for Public Health," Preventing Chronic Disease, Public Health Research, Practice and Policy, Volume 3: No. 2, April 2006. Center for Disease Control:
   https://www.cdc.gov/pcd/issues/2006/apr/05_0167.htm

7. Graedon, Joe, Where Can I Find A List of Anticholinergic Drugs?, PeoplesPharmacy.com,
   https://www.peoplespharmacy.com/2017/05/04/where-can-i-find-a-list-of-anticholinergic-drugs/

8. Risacher, S.L., B.C. McDonald, E.F. Tallman, J.D. West, M.R. Farlow, F.W. Unverzagt, S. Gao, M. Boustani, P.K. Crane, R.C. Petersen, C.R. Jack, Jr., W.J. Jaqust, P.S. Aisen, M.W. Weiner, A.J. Saykin, *Association Between Anticholinergic Medication Use and Cognition, Brain Metabolism, and Brain Atrophy in Cognitively Normal Older Adults*, JAMA Neurology, 2016 Jun 1, 73(6):721-32. Archived on Pubmed.gov.

9. Jongstra, Susan, W.A. van Gool, E.P. Moll van Charante, J.W. van Dalen, L.S.M. Eurlings, E. Richard S.A. Ligthart, *Improving Prediction of Dementia in Primary Care*, Annals of Family Medicine, Vol. 16, No. 3, May/June 2018, 206-210.
   www.annfammed.org http://www.annfammed.org/content/16/3/206.full

10. *Dementia Robs Bilinguals of Second Language First*, Japan Times, May 21, 2013

11. Murphy, David, Aedin Ni Loingsigh, Ingeborg Birnie, Thomas H Bak, *Bilingualism and Dementia: How Some Patients Lose Their Second Language and Rediscover Their First*, The Conversation, November 11, 2019. http://theconversation.com/bilingualism-and-dementia-how-some-patients-lose-their-second-language-and-rediscover-their-first-126631

12. Murphy, David, Aedin Ni Loingsigh, Ingeborg Birnie, Thomas H. Bak, *Bilingualism and Dementia: How Some Patients Lose Their Second Language and Rediscover Their First*, The Conversation, November 11, 2019. http://theconversation.com/bilingualism-and-dementia-how-some-patients-lose-their-second-language-and-rediscover-their-first-126631

13. Bourgeois, Michelle S, *Memory Books and Other Graphic Cuing Systems, Practical Communication and Memory Aids for Adults with Dementia*, Baltimore, Health Professions Press, 2007. Page 16.

14. Murphy, David, Aedin Ni Loingsigh, Ingeborg Birnie, Thomas H Bak, *Bilingualism and Dementia: How Some Patients Lose Their Second Language and Rediscover Their First*, The Conversation, November 11, 2019. http://theconversation.com/bilingualism-and-dementia-how-some-patients-lose-thcir-second-language-and-rediscover-their-first-126631

15. Grimbly, Susan, *English. Please translate?*, Alzlive.com, https://alzlive.com/resources/community/alzheimers-information-languages/

16. Social Care Institute for Excellence, https://www.scie.org.uk/dementia/living-with-dementia/sensory-loss/deafness.asp

17. Young, Alys, Emma Ferguson-Coleman, John Keady, *Understanding Dementia: Effective Information Access from the Deaf Community's Perspective*, Health Social Care in the Community. 2016 January, 24(1):39-47. https://onlinelibrary.wiley.com/doi/abs/10.1111/hsc.12181

18. Young, Alys, Emma Ferguson-Coleman, John Keady, *Understanding the personhood of Deaf people with dementia: Methodological Issues*, Journal of Aging Studies 31 (2014) 62-69. https://www.sciencedirect.com/science/article/pii/S0890406514000486

19. Brown, Steve, *Deaf Interpreter Rupert Dubler on His Role During the Coronavirus Crisis*, https://www.wbur.org/news/2020/04/17/rupert-dubler-asl-interpreter-baker

20. Betz, ME, J. Jones, D.B. Carr, *System facilitators and barriers to discussing older driver safety in primary care settings*, Injury Prevention, August 23, 2015. Archived on Pubmed.gov.

21. Brackey, Jolene, *Creating Moments of Joy Along the Alzheimer's Journey, Fifth Edition*, West Lafayette, Purdue University Press, 2017. Pages 30-32.

22. Bourgeois, Michelle S, *Memory Books and Other Graphic Cuing Systems, Practical Communication and Memory Aids for Adults with Dementia*, Baltimore, Health Professions Press, 2007.

23. Bourgeois, Michelle S, *Memory Books and Other Graphic Cuing Systems, Practical Communication and Memory Aids for Adults with Dementia*, Baltimore, Health Professions Press, 2007. Page 16.

24. Bourgeois, Michelle S, *Memory Books and Other Graphic Cuing Systems, Practical Communication and Memory Aids for Adults with Dementia*, Baltimore, Health Professions Press, 2007. Page 16.

25. Brackey, Jolene, *Creating Moments of Joy Along the Alzheimer's Journey, Fifth Edition*, West Lafayette, Purdue University Press, 2017. Page 108.

26. Scott, Paula Spencer, *Surviving Alzheimer's, Practical Tips and Soul-Saving Wisdom for Caregivers*, Second Edition, San Francisco, Eva Birch Media, 2018. Page 23.

27. Scott, Paula Spencer, *Surviving Alzheimer's, Practical Tips and Soul-Saving Wisdom for Caregivers*, Second Edition, San Francisco, Eva Birch Media, 2018. Page 39

28. Alzheimer's Association, *2019 Alzheimer's Disease Facts and Figures*, page 64.

29. Scott, Paula Spencer, *Surviving Alzheimer's, Practical Tips and Soul-Saving Wisdom for Caregivers*, Second Edition, San Francisco, Eva Birch Media, 2018. Pages 343-346.

30. Ma, Daqing, *Why Do Older People Develop Dementia After Surgery?*, Alzheimer's Society, Great Britain,
https://www.alzheimers.org.uk/research/our-research/research-projects/why-do-older-people-develop-dementia-after-surgery

31. Lin, Frank R., E.J. Metter, R.J. O'Brien, S.M. Resnick, A.B. Zonderman, L. Ferrucci, *Hearing Loss and Incident Dementia*, Archive of Neurology, February 2011; 68(2): 214-20. Archived on Pubmed.gov.

32. Center for Disease Control,
https://www.cdc.gov/disasters/winter/staysafe/hypothermia.html

33. Center for Disease Control,
https://www.cdc.gov/stroke/signs_symptoms.htm

34. Center for Disease Control,
https://www.cdc.gov/stroke/signs_symptoms.htm

35. Coste, Joanne Koenig, *Learning to Speak Alzheimer's, A Groundbreaking Approach for Everyone Dealing with the Disease*, New York, Houghton Mifflin Company, 2003. Pages 62-63.

36. Coste, Joanne Koenig, *Learning to Speak Alzheimer's, A Groundbreaking Approach for Everyone Dealing with the Disease*, New York, Houghton Mifflin Company, 2003. Page 62-63.

37. Cronin-Golomb, A., R. Sugiura, S. Corking, JH Growdon, *Incomplete Achromatopsia in Alzheimer's Disease,* Neurobiology of Aging, 1993 Sept-Oct; 14(5):471-1. Archived on Pubmed.gov.

38. Cronin-Golomb, A., R. Sugiura, S. Corking, JH Growdon, *Incomplete Achromatopsia in Alzheimer's Disease,* Neurobiology of Aging, 1993 Sept-Oct; 14(5):471-1. Archived on Pubmed.gov.

39. Coste, Joanne Koenig, *Learning to Speak Alzheimer's, A Groundbreaking Approach for Everyone Dealing with the Disease*, New York, Houghton Mifflin Company, 2003. Pages 63-65.

40. Calkins, Margaret P. 2002. *How Colour Throws Light on Design in Dementia Care,* Journal of Dementia Care 10 (4): 20-23.

41. Coste, Joanne Koenig, *Learning to Speak Alzheimer's, A Groundbreaking Approach for Everyone Dealing with the Disease*, New York, Houghton Mifflin Company, 2003. Page 65.

42. Coste, Joanne Koenig, *Learning to Speak Alzheimer's, A Groundbreaking Approach for Everyone Dealing with the Disease*, New York, Houghton Mifflin Company, 2003. Pages 87-89.

43. Medicare.gov/coverage/therapeutic-shoes-or-inserts.html.

44. Lin, Frank R., E.J. Metter, R.J. O'Brien, S.M. Rsenick, A.B. Zonderman, L. Ferrucci, *Hearing Loss and Incident Dementia*, Archive of Neurology, February 2011; 68(2): 214-20. Archived on Pubmed.gov.

45. Social Care Institute for Excellence, *Dementia-Friendly Environments: Noise levels*, https://www.scie.org.uk/dementia/supporting-people-with-dementia/dementia-friendly-environments/noise.asp

46. Bushdid, C., M.O. Magnasco, L.B Vosshall, & A. Keller, *Humans Can Discriminate More than 1 Trillion Olfactory Stimuli*, Science 343, 1370–1372 (2014). Archived on Pubmed.gov.

47. Morrison, J., *Human Nose Can Detect 1 Trillion Odours*, Nature, International Weekly Journal of Science, March 20, 2014. https://www.nature.com/news/human-nose-can-detect-1-trillion-odours-1.14904#/b1

232

48. Wasserman, Michael, Simon Atkins, Mark Edwin Kunik, Mary Kenan, Patricia Burkhart Smith, *Alzheimer's and Dementia for Dummies, A Wiley Brand*, Hoboken, John Wiley & Sons, Inc., 2016. Page 150.

49. Scales, K., S. Zimmerman, S.J. Miller, *Evidence-Based Nonpharmacological Practices to Address Behavioral and Psychological Symptoms of Dementia*, Gerontologist, January 2018; 58 (supplement_1):S88-S102. Archived on Pubmed.gov.

50. Brackey, Jolene, *Creating Moments of Joy Along the Alzheimer's Journey, Fifth Edition*, West Lafayette, Purdue University Press, 2017. Pages 68-69.

51. Mace, Nancy L., Peter V. Rabins, *The 36-Hour Day, A Family Guide to Caring for People Who Have Alzheimer Disease, Other Dementias, and Memory Loss*, Sixth Edition, Baltimore, Johns Hopkins University Press, 2017. Pages 152.

52. Brackey, Jolene, *Creating Moments of Joy Along the Alzheimer's Journey, Fifth Edition*, West Lafayette, Purdue University Press, 2017. Page 81.

53. Scott, Paula Spencer, *Surviving Alzheimer's, Practical Tips and Soul-Saving Wisdom for Caregivers*, Second Edition, San Francisco, Eva Birch Media, 2018. Page 178.

54. Scott, Paula Spencer, *Surviving Alzheimer's, Practical Tips and Soul-Saving Wisdom for Caregivers*, Second Edition, San Francisco, Eva Birch Media, 2018. Pages 167-168.

55. Coste, Joanne Koenig, *Learning to Speak Alzheimer's, A Groundbreaking Approach for Everyone Dealing with the Disease*, New York, Houghton Mifflin Company, 2003. Pages 119-121.

56. Mace, Nancy L., Peter V. Rabins, *The 36-Hour Day, A Family Guide to Caring for People Who Have Alzheimer Disease, Other Dementias, and Memory Loss*, Sixth Edition, Baltimore, Johns Hopkins University Press, 2017. Pages 170-171.

57. Wasserman, Michael, Simon Atkins, Mark Edwin Kunik, Mary Kenan, Patricia Burkhart Smith, *Alzheimer's and Dementia for Dummies, A Wiley Brand*, Hoboken, John Wiley & Sons, Inc., 2016. Page 31.

58. Mertens, Brian, Susan B. Sorenson, *Current Considerations About the Elderly and Firearms*, American Journal of Public Health, March 2012; Volume 102(3), 396-400. Archived on the U.S. National Library of Medicine, National Institutes of Health website: https://www.ncbi.nlm.nih.gov/pmc/articles/PMC3487668/

59. Brackey, Jolene, *Creating Moments of Joy Along the Alzheimer's Journey, Fifth Edition*, West Lafayette, Purdue University Press, 2017. Page 199.

60. Brackey, Jolene, *Creating Moments of Joy Along the Alzheimer's Journey, Fifth Edition*, West Lafayette, Purdue University Press, 2017. Page 198-203.

61. Brackey, Jolene, *Creating Moments of Joy Along the Alzheimer's Journey, Fifth Edition*, West Lafayette, Purdue University Press, 2017. Page 198-203.

62. Mace, Nancy L., Peter V. Rabins, *The 36-Hour Day, A Family Guide to Caring for People Who Have Alzheimer Disease, Other Dementias, and Memory Loss*, Sixth Edition, Baltimore, Johns Hopkins University Press, 2017. Pages 100.

63. Kidney & Urology Foundation of America, Inc., *Urodynamic Testing*, http://www.kidneyurology.org/Library/Urologic_Health.php/Urodynamic_Testing.php

64. Mace, Nancy L., Peter V. Rabins, *The 36-Hour Day, A Family Guide to Caring for People Who Have Alzheimer Disease, Other Dementias, and Memory Loss*, Sixth Edition, Baltimore, Johns Hopkins University Press, 2017. Page 265-267.

65. Mace, Nancy L., Peter V. Rabins, *The 36-Hour Day, A Family Guide to Caring for People Who Have Alzheimer Disease, Other Dementias, and Memory Loss*, Sixth Edition, Baltimore, Johns Hopkins University Press, 2017. Page 101.

66. National Institute on Aging: https://www.nia.nih.gov/news/number-alzheimers-deaths-found-be-underreported (accessed 1/28/2019).

67. Snow, Teepa, Senior Helpers, "Understanding Dementia Care," *The Ten Early Signs of Dementia*, YouTube, July 23, 2013. https://www.youtube.com/watch?v=pqmqC-702Yg4

68. Dunne, T.E., S.A. Neargarder, P.B. Cipolloni, A. Cronin-Golomb, *Visual Contrast Enhances Food and Liquid Intake in Advanced Alzheimer's Disease*, Clinical Nutrition, 2004, Aug; 23(4):533-8. Archived on Pubmed.gov.

69. Cronin-Golomb, Alice, *Cognitive Problems, Sensory Abilities*, Posit Science, BrainHQ.com https://www.brainhq.com/brain-resources/brain-plasticity/brain-plasticity-luminaries/alice-cronin-golomb-phd

70. National Institutes of Health (NIH), https://www.nia.nih.gov/news/number-alzheimers-deaths-found-be-underreported

71. Kohn, Robert, Wendy Verhoek-Oftedahl, *Caregiving and Elder Abuse*, National Institutes of Health, Medical Health Review Issue 2011 Feb; 94(2): 47-49. Archived on https://www.ncbi.nlm.nih.gov/pmc/articles/PMC4961478/

72. Gilles, Gary, LCPC, *Addressing Caregiver Stress to Prevent Elder Abuse*, Mentalhelp.net, https://www.mentalhelp.net/blogs/addressing-caregiver-stress-to-prevent-elder-abuse/

73. Schempp, Donna, *Emotional Side of Caregiving*, Family Caregiver Alliance, 2014. Archived on https://www.caregiver.org/emotional-side-caregiving

74. Schempp, Donna, *Emotional Side of Caregiving*, Family Caregiver Alliance, 2014. Archived on https://www.caregiver.org/emotional-side-caregiving

75. Scott, Paula Spencer, *Surviving Alzheimer's, Practical Tips and Soul-Saving Wisdom for Caregivers*, Second Edition, San Francisco, Eva Birch Media, 2018. Pages 342-346.

76. Scott, Paula Spencer, *Surviving Alzheimer's, Practical Tips and Soul-Saving Wisdom for Caregivers*, Second Edition, San Francisco, Eva Birch Media, 2018. Page 349.

77. Scott, Paula Spencer, *Surviving Alzheimer's, Practical Tips and Soul-Saving Wisdom for Caregivers*, Second Edition, San Francisco, Eva Birch Media, 2018. Pages 342-346.

78. Scott, Paula Spencer, *Surviving Alzheimer's, Practical Tips and Soul-Saving Wisdom for Caregivers*, Second Edition, San Francisco, Eva Birch Media, 2018. Pages 342-346.

79. Simmons, Kevin M., *Suicides and Death with Dignity*, Journal of Law and the Biosciences, 2018 August; 5(2): 436-439. Archived on https://www.ncbi.nlm.nih.gov/pmc/articles/PMC6121057/

80. Dementia Care Central, *Alzheimer's / Dementia Care Costs: Home Care, Adult Day Care, Assisted Living & Nursing Homes*, https://www.dementiacarecentral.com/assisted-living-home-care-costs/

81. Famakinwa, Joyce, *Despite High Costs CCRC at Home Models are Gaining Traction*, Home Healthcare News, December 2, 2019, https://homehealthcarenews.com/2019/12/despite-high-costs-ccrc-at-home-models-gaining-traction/

82. Huntsberry-Lett, Ashley, *End-of-Life Care: Signs That Death is Near*, Aging Care, https://www.agingcare.com/articles/end-of-life-care-signs-that-death-is-near-443741.htm

83. Scott, Paula Spencer, *Surviving Alzheimer's, Practical Tips and Soul-Saving Wisdom for Caregivers*, Second Edition, San Francisco, Eva Birch Media, 2018. Pages 363-365.

84. Scott, Paula Spencer, *Surviving Alzheimer's, Practical Tips and Soul-Saving Wisdom for Caregivers*, Second Edition, San Francisco, Eva Birch Media, 2018. Pages 339-346.

85. Heiser, K. Gabriel, *Filial Responsibility Laws and Medicaid*, Medicaid Secrets, Aging Care, https://www.agingcare.com/articles/filial-responsibility-and-medicaid-197746.htm

86. United States Government, *Four Tips to Find Unclaimed Money.* Archived on https://www.usa.gov/unclaimed-money

87. Ianzito, Christina, *More Drugstores Take Back Your Unused Meds*, AARP, June 18, 2018, https://www.aarp.org/health/drugs-supplements/info-2018/drug-stores-medication-disposal.html

Recommended Reading

If you can only buy one other reference book, then I recommend *The 36-Hour Day, A Family Guide to Caring for People Who Have Alzheimer's Disease, Other Dementias, and Memory Loss*, by Nancy Mace, MA and Peter V. Rabin, MD, MPH, now in its sixth edition. It was originally published in 1981 and remains a go-to reference on the subject of memory loss for people like you and me.

If you are interested in additional reading material, this is what's on my bookshelf:

Brackey, Jolene, *Creating Moments of Joy Along the Alzheimer's Journey, Fifth Edition*, West Lafayette, Purdue University Press, 2017

Bredesen, Dale E., *The End of Alzheimer's, The First Program to Prevent and Reverse Cognitive Decline*, New York, Avery, an imprint of Penguin Random House, 2017

Bourgeois, Michelle S, *Memory Books and Other Graphic Cuing Systems, Practical Communication and Memory Aids for Adults with Dementia*, Baltimore, Health Professions Press, 2007.

Capossela, Cappy, Sheila Warnock, *Share the Care, How to Organize a Group to Care for Someone Who is Seriously Ill*, New York, Fireside, 2004.

Coste, Joanne Koenig, *Learning to Speak Alzheimer's, A Groundbreaking Approach for Everyone Dealing with the Disease*, New York, Houghton Mifflin Company, 2003.

Goodheart, Annette, *Laughter Therapy, How to Laugh About Everything in Your Life That Isn't Really Funny*, Santa Barbara, Less Stress Press, 1994.

Petersen, Barry, *Jan's Story*, Lake Forest, Behler Publications, LLC, 2010.

Scott, Paula Spencer, *Surviving Alzheimer's, Practical Tips and Soul-Saving Wisdom for Caregivers*, Second Edition, San Francisco, Eva Birch Media, 2018.

Shagam, Janet Yagoda, *An Unintended Journey, A Caregiver's Guide to Dementia*, New York, Prometheus Books, 2013.

Wasserman, Michael, Simon Atkins, Mark Edwin Kunik, Mary Kenan, Patricia Burkhart Smith, *Alzheimer's and Dementia for Dummies, A Wiley Brand*, Hoboken, John Wiley & Sons, Inc., 2016.

If you organized a group for Alzheimer's play dates, these are the books on my bookshelf:

Bell, Virginia, David Troxel, Tonya M. Cox, and Robin Hamon, *The Best Friends Book of Alzheimer's Activities, Vol 1*, Baltimore, Health Professions Press, 2004.
— *The Best Friends Book of Alzheimer's Activities, Vol 2*, Baltimore, Health Professions Press, 2008.

238

Index

About the Author

Tracy Cram Perkins's twelve years of caregiving for her parents with dementia and an uncle with mild dementia created the base for *Dementia Home Care, How to Prepare Before, During, and After.*

Caring for her family, she learned firsthand the depression, anxiety, and guilt that comes with dementia care and how each person's journey follows a different path. She found laughter is an important part of surviving caregiving.

She's a Halloween fanatic who creates humorous tombstones like "Viagra, the Fifth Hour" for her display. Despite what her neighbors think, the only bodies in her graveyard at Halloween are the moles who insist her front yard is a mole recycling center. Try as she might, she can't convince them to go into the light.

Tracy and her husband reside on Washington State's Olympic Peninsula. They share a home with assorted fish and two cats, Ax and Dently, who demand their obedience between naps.

You can find out more about Tracy's upcoming books, sign up to her mailing list to receive *10 Steps to Calming Aggressive Dementia Behavior*, or get in touch with Tracy at her website: ***TRACYCRAMPERKINS.COM.***

Finally, please consider leaving a review online if you enjoyed this book. Even if it is only a line or two, it will help get the word out.

More Ways to Contact Tracy:

Email: tracy@tracycramperkins.com

Blog: tracycramperkins.com/home/blog/

Facebook: Tracy Cram Perkins, Author